O.W.N.E.R

THE MIND MOUTH BODY CONNECTION

SHEREE WERTZ

Core Message: You are the O.W.N.E.R. The 5 Pillars of Optimal Health:

- **O**xygen
- **W**ater
- **N**utrition
- **E**nough sleep
- **R**especting your one body

Your Health is Your Greatest Investment

You get one body; your body is the vehicle that carries you through life.

Shift your habits and live not only longer but healthier. The goal of this book will focus on empowering individuals to take ownership of their health by understanding the interconnectedness of their thoughts, beliefs, mindset, mouth and body. This book emphasizes the importance of prevention, personalized care and the critical role of oral health as a window to overall well being.

Table of Contents

Disclaimer

This book was written to provide general information and education between the reader and the author and should not be used for diagnosis or treatment. It is not a substitute for professional medical advice, diagnosis or treatment. Consult your healthcare provider for any medical advice or other related questions and do not avoid treatment based on reading this book. What was written at the time of publication may change with further research and evolution of life as we know it.

Anyone who embarks on a holistic healing journey involving dietary, habit and lifestyle changes accepts full responsibility for their decisions.

As someone with dyslexia, I find large paragraphs challenging to read. So, this book is structured the way I prefer to read: with spacing clear, concise, and easy to navigate. With the support of family, friends, and AI, I've crafted it to be both accessible and engaging.

Some of the products discussed may be an affiliate link, unless you use a specific link we provide with a code, we are not compensated for recommendations. We recommend that you do your own independent research before using or purchasing anything.

Acknowledgements

To my parents, who taught me the value of hard work, determination, and belief in myself. Your courage, love, and unwavering support have shaped me in countless ways. Thank you, Mom, for proofreading and typing my endless edits, and Dad, for teaching me to persevere, "don't talk about it, just do it."

To my sister, for always having my back, even when I didn't know I needed it. Your unwavering support means the world to me.

To my beautiful daughter: from the moment I heard your heartbeat, I knew our bond was unbreakable. Your unconditional love and the joys of motherhood have taught me patience, humility, and the beauty of loving unapologetically.

To Mike, for reminding me to take my own advice and keeping me nourished when I was too focused to pause thank you for being my rock.

To my family, friends, and patients: your trust in me to guide you on your health journeys has been an honor. You inspire me every day, and I deeply appreciate each of you.

To anyone holding back on a dream: go for it. The world needs your unique gift. Thank you, Marie Forleo, for reminding me that "everything is figureoutable."

To Russell Brunson, Steve Larsen, and Marly Jaxx: your guidance showed me new ways to share my mission and stay resilient. To Andy Griffith, my sounding board and tech support through life's toughest moments—thank you for helping me keep moving forward.

To you, the reader: I am humbled and grateful that you chose this book amidst countless options. May it empower you to make informed choices for a healthier, happier life.

As a thank-you, I've included free resources and a workbook to help you take action as you read. Visit www.shereewertz.com/owner-resources to access them.

Foreword

We live in an era where health advice is everywhere, scroll your social media, turn on the TV, or walk down the aisle of any bookstore, and you'll find yourself drowning in conflicting information. Eat this, not that. Breathe this way. Sleep more, but hustle harder. It's overwhelming, isn't it?

This book is here to cut through that noise.

Now, more than ever, we're realizing how interconnected our bodies are. Science is confirming what many of us have felt all along. Health isn't about quick fixes or isolated symptoms. It's about the whole picture, the whole body, working together in harmony.

But here's the catch: the answers aren't always in the headlines. They're in the basics. The fundamentals. The things we've overlooked in the chaos of modern living. Breathing deeply, drinking water, eating nourishing food, sleeping enough, and honoring the incredible machine that is your body.

I wrote this book because I've lived it. I've seen what happens when health takes a backseat personally, as a mom, and through decades of experience in the dental field. I've battled breast cancer, rebuilt my life, and stood at the crossroads of despair and hope. Every time the path back to health both physical and emotional started with the basics.

This book isn't about giving you another long to-do list. It's about helping you connect the dots. Your health isn't just about one thing; it's about *everything* working together. And it starts in a place you might not expect, your mouth.

Yes, your mouth is a window into your overall health. How you breathe, how you eat, how you sleep, and how you care for your oral health can transform not just your body but your life.

Together, we're going to unpack what's normal versus what's common, break down myths, and build a framework that empowers you to take ownership of your health. No gimmicks, no fads, just real, actionable insights to help you thrive.

The time to take charge is now. Not when illness strikes or exhaustion sets in. But today, while you have the power to make small, impactful changes that ripple through every part of your life.

This book is my invitation to you. Your health is your greatest asset, and you are its sole owner. Let's unlock the knowledge, tools, and mindset you need to protect it, grow it, and invest in a lifetime of returns.

Sheree

CHAPTER 1

Wake Up Call, Welcome and Purpose

Cells can heal themselves when they become unhealthy. The moment I realized I wasn't in control of my health was the day I found myself sitting in a sterile doctor's office, staring at a diagnosis I didn't expect. My heart raced as I replayed years of neglect skipped workouts, drive through takeout, and stress-filled days with little sleep. I thought I was too busy to focus on my well-being. But in reality, I was too distracted to notice my health slipping away.

That moment was my wake-up call.

But here's the good news: it doesn't take a crisis to start taking control. In fact, the sooner you begin, the better your chances of thriving not just surviving in today's fast-paced world. This book is your guide to reclaiming the reins of your health, one decision at a time.

Your body has an incredible capacity to heal itself. If you are injured or become ill your body should quickly and efficiently deal with the problem and restore itself to health. Cells can heal themselves when they become unhealthy and replicate to replace destroyed or damaged cells. In fact, our bodies are in a constant state of removing damage and producing new, healthy tissue. Our immune system is also meant to deal with intruders such as viruses, bacteria, and toxins.

Why then, if our bodies are so well designed, are 20.4% of American adults dealing with chronic pain and more than 40% of Americans are affected by chronic diseases?

Many factors inhibit a body's natural self-healing functions. Some are obvious, and others we are still learning about. We do know that your body needs adequate uninterrupted sleep, clean water, healthy foods, and exercise. Various types of stress and toxins cause harm. Even your mindset can impact your health.

You don't know what you don't know. The system is changing little by little as we are finally realizing what we have been doing is not working. There are people taking a new look at a lot of things. There is so much information at our fingertips. We live in an era of information overload, work overload and sugar overload. Even with all the knowledge we do have, there are still millions of people suffering from all sorts of chronic illnesses, along with snoring, clenching, grinding, and not sleeping. Six out of 10 people are taking pills that are treating symptoms affecting their quality of life. Something needs to change.

The Greatest Investment You'll Ever Make - YOU

Imagine waking up every day with the energy to do what you love, the clarity to make decisions confidently, and the resilience to face life's challenges head-on. Now, picture the opposite a constant struggle with fatigue, stress, lack of sleep, and a growing list of medical bills that seem to control your every move.

For many of us, the latter feels far too familiar. And yet, in a world flooded with health advice, supplements, and quick fixes, we often miss the most important message: **you are the owner of your health**.

The truth is, we're living in a time where personal health ownership isn't just important it's essential. With rising chronic illnesses, unpredictable healthcare systems, and the overwhelming influence of modern lifestyles, the responsibility for our well-being has shifted squarely onto our shoulders. No one else is better equipped to protect your body, mind, and future than you.

In this book, we'll explore why owning your health is not just a trend but a necessity. We'll uncover practical ways to take charge, empowering you to become the CEO of your own well-being.

Because if there's one investment that pays dividends for the rest of your life it's your health.

As a Mom and dental hygienist, I did not know a lot. We know the connection the mouth has to the rest of the body, but it is still overlooked when we talk about overall health and wellness. The more I learn, the more I realize I don't know. We live in two ecosystems, one outside our body and one inside our body.

When our autonomic nervous system senses we are in danger, it takes us out of the thrive state and puts us in fight-or-flight state. Most people operate from this state more than not. The mouth and tongue play an integral role in why we are not meeting our basic needs.

When I first started to write this book, cavities were the #1 preventable childhood diseases, and I wanted to change that. I worked for a mobile dental company and saw how many kids were affected. I was shocked. I was taught we need to teach our patients about our **BFF** with a **DD:**

- **B**rush
- **F**loss
- Use **F**luoride toothpaste
- Be intentional with your **D**iet
- Visit your **D**entist twice a year

If that is true, why have cavities been the #1 preventable childhood disease for decades? Even with all the knowledge and technology we have, it is worse now than when I graduated over 30 years ago. I now understand cavities are a warning sign our body is out of balance, and breathing is where we should start if we truly want to be healthy.

This book is some of what I did know, but mostly what I wish I had known before my daughter was born. It would have made things so much easier, and maybe I would have not felt like I was failing as a dental hygienist and at parenting.

What I found in trying to help my own daughter was that we as a society are struggling to meet even our basic needs. Maslow's theory of hierarchy states we must meet those needs before we can move up the pyramid. This is where O.W.N.E.R. was created.

I have learned so much as a Mom. The biggest thing is **Trust Your Instincts**, they are never wrong!

"What you believe to be true is true," you hear it all the time.

Your thoughts really do create your reality, be conscious of your thoughts. Everything starts from the head down.

I decided to be the change that I want to see in the world of healthcare. I now have the confidence to know that my knowledge was just as valuable as anyone's. I had a patient say, "You made a difference to me. Please share what you know."

It is funny because my mom always said, "Once you get in your 50s, you no longer care what people think." Well, she was right about that! I now realize it does not matter if everyone agrees with you. Someone needs what you have to offer; you owe it to the world to share your message and knowledge.

Welcome And Purpose

This is your time to align with yourself and step into your power. You deserve a life that lights you up. You can have it all if you choose to claim it! Say yes to becoming the best version of yourself. Choose empowering thoughts, uplifting feelings, and actions that align with your vision. Remember, every moment is a chance to begin again.

Your mindset shapes your reality, and choosing to do what makes you happy is one of the most powerful decisions you can make. Too often, we hold ourselves back because of limiting beliefs or societal expectations that tell us happiness is selfish or unattainable. But the truth is, when you prioritize joy and align your life with what truly fulfills you, everything else begins to fall into place. A positive mindset empowers you to let go of what you've been taught to believe and embrace what feels right for *you*. Happiness isn't a luxury it's a necessity for your health, relationships, and overall well-being. Remember, when you choose happiness, you show up as your best self, and that energy has the power to inspire everyone around you.

Self-care isn't optional it's essential. Yet in today's fast-paced world, we often take our bodies for granted, pushing through fatigue, stress, or pain until it's too late. Ignoring these signals compromises our long-term health, well-being, and overall quality of life.

- Lifelong Responsibility: You can't trade in your body, so preserving it is a lifelong commitment. The care you give today ensures vitality for the future.
- Choices Shape Health: Your daily habits, how you eat, sleep, move, and manage stress, create your health over time. Positive habits build strength; neglect erodes it.

- Listen to Your Body: Signals like snoring, clenching, grinding, getting up in the middle of the night to pee, bleeding gums, pain, fatigue, or burnout are your body's way of asking for care. Pay attention and respond.
- Holistic Care: True health isn't just physical. Mental, emotional, and physical well-being are deeply connected. Your mindset shapes your satisfaction and overall health.

This book is here to guide you in honoring, nourishing, and listening to your body. Through simple shifts, better breathing, restorative sleep, and a foundation for lifelong oral and systemic health you'll gain tools to improve not just your life, but the lives of your loved ones.

Why This Matters

Our healthcare system is often more focused on treating symptoms than creating true health. It's time to ask better questions and seek better answers. When you align with yourself and listen to your body, you reclaim the power to shape your own health. Be satisfied with where you are while staying eager for more.

The basics matter. This book starts with the fundamental needs of your body: balance, nourishment, and attention. Whether you're planning for pregnancy, improving your oral health, or simply looking for ways to thrive, this book will help you ask the right questions and take actionable steps.

Your mouth is a window to your body. No pain doesn't mean no problem, it's giving you signals. Learn what to look for, how to listen, and how to take action.

The best time to start is now, wherever you are in your journey. It's never too late to give your body what it needs to thrive. Together, we'll explore how small, consistent changes can make a profound difference in your life.

Values and Beliefs

I am a huge believer that our own thoughts, values and beliefs impact our decisions. Most thoughts are generational, they started with what our parents' thoughts and beliefs were, and what their parents taught them, and so on are passed down.

Those beliefs impact the value we place on everything. They impact whether we even go to a doctor or dentist for treatment in the first place.

They impact the choices we make. If you choose to go to a doctor or dentist and do not agree with what they are saying, you have the right to refuse treatment. Do your research and find a provider that is in line with your beliefs.

I am a dental hygienist. My ex-husband was a dentist, my father-in-law was an orthodontist, and our daughter wore braces three times and had a sleep breathing issue related to her tongue function. We were not taught to look at breathing or tongue function and had no idea that improper tongue function and habits were responsible for changing the position of her teeth once her braces were removed.

Keep in mind that each doctor, dentist and provider will have their own belief system based on their experiences in life which affects the way they establish their practice. It is not fair for you to dictate what treatment the doctor or dentist provides if it is not in line with their beliefs. Find a different provider if you are not meshing.

Picking the right provider is key to a mutually respectful relationship.

Finding a provider is like dating! It may take kissing a few frogs before you find the right one. I have seen posts on social media that say don't trust a person who offers this or that.

You get to make informed decisions about your mouth and your body for overall health that are in line with your personal belief system and not just take someone else's word. Learn to be your own advocate and trust your gut and your instincts.

You are right, more often than not. Trust yourself!!

How to Use This Book

This book is designed to guide you step by step on your journey toward better health. Each chapter builds upon the previous one, showing how every element connects to form a complete picture.

Here's how to get the most out of it:

- Focus on What You Can Control: Prioritize areas where you can make immediate changes.
- Take Action: Use the steps and resources provided to implement new habits.
- Go at Your Own Pace: Make adjustments that feel right for you this is your journey.
- Trust Your Instincts: Listen to your body and intuition as you navigate your health path.

While reading the book straight through provides a comprehensive understanding of the big picture, you can also skip to the sections that resonate most with your current needs. This flexibility ensures the book meets you where you are.

Why I Wrote This Book

This book is the resource I wish I had when I began my health journey. Inside, you'll find actionable steps, additional resources, and guidance on specific topics. If you'd like to dive deeper, I also offer a course that expands on these principles. For more information or to work with me directly, visit www.shereewertz.com.

A Note on Language

To keep the flow natural, I've chosen to use pronouns like "I," "we," "your," and "our." These shifts in tone reflect the personal and collaborative nature of this book.

My Hope for You

My goal is to change the way you view your health starting with your mouth. By understanding its profound connection to the rest of your body, you'll see how small habit shifts can create big changes.

Sometimes, achieving optimal health requires a team of professionals. I'll guide you on when to seek help and what to look for in the right provider. But ultimately, this journey is about you. Becoming the O.W.N.E.R. of your health means embracing the process and empowering yourself with knowledge.

The Book's Mission

This book's mission is to help you take control of your health by providing tools, insights, and actionable steps. Knowledge is a powerful catalyst for change, and the more you know, the better choices you can make.

True health starts from the top down, your mind, your thoughts, your breathing, and how you care for the one body you have. You are your greatest asset, and investing in yourself is the key to living your best life.

A Perspective Shift

It's easy to ignore what we don't understand. I know because I did the same. But when I realized I was only hurting myself, I changed my perspective and that shift created the most significant transformation in my life.

If this resonates with you, remember this truth: What you don't change, you choose.

Be the O.W.N.E.R. You Are

Your health is your responsibility. Meeting your basic needs is the foundation for thriving, not just surviving. This book is here to support you as you take the reins and become the O.W.N.E.R. of your life.

Let's get started.

CHAPTER 2

Introduction: The Foundation of Health

To truly unlock lasting health, it's important to understand three foundational concepts that will be woven throughout this book. These ideas while powerful on their own are interconnected and form the basis of the O.W.N.E.R. framework.

The Power of Your Thoughts

Our thoughts are more powerful than we often realize. They shape how we view the world, how we respond to challenges, and even how our body functions at a cellular level. As we discuss the foundation of health, it's essential to understand the profound connection between mindset and well-being. Your beliefs and perceptions don't just influence your emotions they influence your biology, too

Everything begins with your thoughts. You have an internal guidance system that considers who you are and your environment. Trust it. Take what resonates with you and leave the rest. Your thoughts and beliefs shape your reality.

I know this firsthand. I've faced miscarriages, cancer, and unimaginable heartache. At 19, I was told I'd never have children due to severe endometriosis. Despite the odds, I held onto my belief that I would one day become a mother. It wasn't easy. I had eight miscarriages and many setbacks but I never stopped believing.

Our thoughts send signals to our bodies. Positive thoughts can heal, while negative ones can harm. Science shows that less than 5% of illnesses are genetic; most are influenced by our environment, habits, and mindset. This is known as epigenetics the idea that we can change how our genes are expressed by changing our thoughts and behaviors.

The Mind-Mouth-Body Connection

Your mouth is more than just where food enters or words are formed; it's a gateway to your entire body's health. Breathing, chewing, and even oral hygiene influence systems like digestion, energy levels, immunity, and mental clarity. This concept, the mind-mouth-body connection, will serve as a cornerstone throughout this book.

In later chapters, you'll learn how this connection ties directly to specific health pillars like proper breathing, hydration, and nutrition.

The Power of Small Changes

Big transformations don't require overwhelming, all-or-nothing changes. In fact, the most profound health shifts come from small, consistent actions. Tiny adjustments in your daily habits like breathing through your nose or drinking an extra glass of water can create a ripple effect, improving your overall well-being in ways you might not expect.

As you move through each pillar of the O.W.N.E.R. framework, you'll see how these small changes fit into the bigger picture of your health journey.

Epigenetics: How Small Actions Influence Big Outcomes

Our thoughts and environment can influence how your genes express themselves. By fostering a mindset of self-love and empowerment, you can create a positive ripple effect on your physical health.

You are not just the sum of your genetic code. Through the field of epigenetics, we've learned that your lifestyle choices, what you eat, how you breathe, and the quality of your sleep have the power to influence how your genes express themselves. In other words, your daily habits can "turn on" or "turn off" certain genetic markers that affect your health outcomes.

Even more fascinating, the choices you make today don't just impact your own health, they can ripple into future generations, shaping the genetic expressions of your children and grandchildren.

This concept of epigenetics will come into focus in later chapters, especially in discussions about nutrition, mindset, and personalized health strategies. For now, it's important to understand this: *Small actions can create big outcomes.* You hold the power to influence your health in ways that go far beyond the moment.

Most people spend their lives chasing wealth, often neglecting their health until a problem arises. I was one of those people. I believed I was healthy watching what I ate, filtering my water, working out, and getting enough sleep until the bottom fell out. A decision by someone else changed everything, shaking my trust in myself, my habits, and my choices.

For years, I stayed busy to avoid facing my feelings. I blamed others, held onto resentment, and struggled to move forward. Eventually, I realized it wasn't about what happened to me; it was about how I chose to respond. I had to face my feelings, forgive myself, and take responsibility for my life. Self-forgiveness was the hardest step, but it was the most freeing.

Prevention is always better than waiting until your body forces you to pay attention. If you feel out of sync, it's time to change your perspective, thoughts, and habits.

Your mouth is a gateway to your overall health, yet it is often overlooked in medical care. Conditions like bleeding gums, cavities, and other dental diseases can signal deeper systemic issues. For instance:

- Bleeding gums can indicate inflammation linked to heart disease, diabetes, or even cancer.
- Mouth breathing contributes to conditions like anxiety, ADHD, and cardiovascular disease.
- Oral health reflects the health of the entire body, yet it is treated separately, even by insurance.

Dental disease is often silent, **no pain doesn't mean no problem.** Listening to your body, paying attention to subtle signs, and addressing oral health early can prevent larger health issues down the road.

The One Body You Have

Growing up, we're often taught to care for material possessions like cars, but not for our own bodies. We maintain cars with gas, oil changes, and regular tune-ups, yet we neglect the one body we'll have for our entire lives. Doesn't it make sense to prioritize ourselves above any replaceable item?

The human body is a complex, interconnected system with 11 major organ systems working together. Traditional healthcare often treats symptoms in isolation, ignoring the synergy between systems. For example, proper breathing impacts sleep, stress levels, and even oral health. By understanding how the body functions as a whole, we can identify root causes, prevent issues, and achieve lasting wellness.

Ask Yourself

Take a moment to reflect on your own health:

- What is your personal health journey?
- How do you feel about your health today?
- Are you experiencing symptoms like pain, fatigue, or stress?
- How is your oral health?
- Has your health impacted your family's well-being?
- Are you listening to your body?

If you're not healthy, it's harder to be there for others. Don't wait for a wake-up call like I did, start now.

The Power of Perception Mindset and Beliefs:

Your perception controls your biology. When people talk about genes "turning on or off," it's really your environment and perception signaling your body to read those genetic blueprints. You are not a victim of your genes.

Have you heard of the placebo effect? It works because a positive belief in healing triggers the body to heal itself. Studies show that one-third of all healing even in surgeries can be attributed to the placebo effect or positive thoughts. Similarly, negative thoughts can harm just as powerfully.

To truly heal and thrive, we need to shift from problem-solving to prevention. Love yourself, believe in your worth, and align your actions with what you want.

The Role of Self-Love and Intuition

Self-love isn't indulgent, it's the foundation of health. Negative emotions are warning signs that something is out of alignment. Pay attention to them. When you feel good, you're on the right path.

For a long time, I ignored my intuition and let others' opinions dictate my life. I wish I had known sooner that my opinion of myself is the only one that truly matters. No one knows you better than you. Trust yourself and listen to your instincts, they're always right.

Looking back, I see how much my thoughts and beliefs influenced my health. After multiple losses, two suicides in my family, and a battle with breast cancer, I realized I had been holding onto anger and replaying negative emotions. This mental state created an environment for disease in my body.

Although it was a challenging time, cancer became a blessing in disguise. It taught me the importance of aligning my thoughts, emotions, and habits to create health rather than disease. I learned that healing begins with self-love, forgiveness, and a commitment to caring for my body.

Takeaways

You are more powerful than you realize. By changing your perspective, beliefs, and habits, you can change your biology and create the life you desire. Your thoughts are the most important tool you have. They can heal you or harm you.

- Choose thoughts that feel good.
- Love yourself unconditionally.
- Trust your instincts and listen to your body.

S.H.I.F.T. System

Simple Habits Incentives For Transformation

Focus: Creating transformational health shifts through small, sustainable habits.

Key Components:

1. **S**mall Steps: Start with manageable changes, like nasal breathing or adding one healthy meal.
2. **H**abits: Build consistency through daily practices like tongue posture checks and hydration.
3. **I**dentify: Identify areas of imbalance (e.g., sleep, nutrition, oral health) and address them.
4. **F**ocus: Prioritize one habit at a time to reduce overwhelm and encourage success.
5. **T**hrive: Cultivate long-term transformation through a system of layered, sustainable habits.

Your health journey is yours alone. Start with small steps, believe in yourself, and remember that happiness is a choice you make every day.

My Mouth Has Always Been an Issue

From infancy, my mouth was a source of challenges. I was a colicky baby, anemic, and frequently had high fevers. I was given liquid iron and Tetracycline, which permanently stained my teeth, leaving them yellow-orange and causing me to feel self-conscious from an early age.

At age five, I had my first traumatic dental experiences. My dentist had a "hand over mouth" approach, silencing fidgeting or squirming with intimidation. It left me terrified of dental visits. Switching to a pediatric dentist at my mom's insistence was a relief, but those early fears stayed with me, exacerbated by the fact that I couldn't breathe comfortably when laid back in the chair, an issue still overlooked in many dental offices.

By age 10, the stains on my teeth had caught the attention of my peers. A boy on my bus made it his mission to ridicule me, nicknaming me "Crusty" and encouraging others to laugh. The bullying crushed my confidence and taught me to hide my smile. It wasn't until I got braces and, later, veneers that I could finally smile without shame.

These early experiences shaped my passion for oral health. I want others to understand how poor oral health can profoundly impact a child's self-esteem, mental health, and overall well-being. In the 1960s, we didn't know the long-term effects of medications like tetracycline. Today, we have the advantage of knowledge to prevent similar issues for the next generation.

The Emotional Impact of Childhood Experiences

Teasing and bullying leave lasting scars. As a child, I didn't know how to process embarrassment and sadness. I repressed my feelings and pretended I was fine, but those emotions resurfaced later in life.

Our generation was taught to "suck it up" and move on, but that approach doesn't address the root of trauma or emotional wounds. As a parent, I've said similar things to my own daughter, but I've learned that when we know better, we can do better. Addressing emotions, listening to feelings, and teaching self-compassion can help break the cycle for future generations.

Finding Purpose Through Passion

High school was when I discovered my love for dentistry. A vocational program in dental assisting opened my eyes to a field where I could help others while learning more about my own oral health. Passion for a subject makes learning enjoyable, and I've been on a lifelong quest for knowledge ever since. The more I learn, the more I realize how interconnected our health is, and how much more there is to explore.

My mission now is to educate parents on how they can support their children's health starting with the mouth. Simple, sustainable habits can ensure their health for years to come.

Happiness and Perspective: The Key to Change

Happiness is a choice, and finding joy in life makes everything flow more smoothly. Negative emotions and resistance often stem from not listening to our instincts or needs. When we align with what feels good and release the need to control or "earn" our worth, life becomes more fulfilling. While this is a simple concept, if you are not in a good mental state, finding happiness can be hard. Emotions can be a spiral you can go up or down, you choose which way they go. It may be impossible to go from powerless to joy, and happy people may be irritating to you depending on where you are at the moment. Start where you are and work up the scale of emotions one thought at a time.

What happened in the past belongs in the past. Reliving it by constantly talking about it doesn't serve you—it only keeps you stuck. I know this from experience. For years, I would tell anyone who would listen, "Can you believe this happened to me?" All it did was reinforce my pain and prevent me from moving forward.

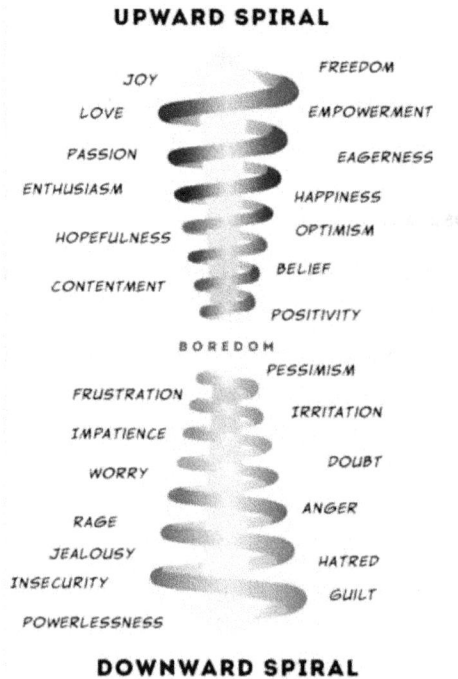

UPWARD SPIRAL

JOY   FREEDOM

LOVE   EMPOWERMENT

PASSION   EAGERNESS

ENTHUSIASM   HAPPINESS

HOPEFULNESS OPTIMISM

CONTENTMENT BELIEF

      POSITIVITY

BOREDOM

      PESSIMISM

FRUSTRATION IRRITATION

IMPATIENCE

WORRY   DOUBT

      ANGER

RAGE

JEALOUSY   HATRED

INSECURITY   GUILT

POWERLESSNESS

DOWNWARD SPIRAL

Other people's actions affected my life plan, and at times, it felt like the rug was pulled out from underneath me repeatedly in a short span. But eventually, I realized I had two choices:

1. Play the victim, stay stuck, and wallow in it.
2. Take the lesson, set boundaries, put myself and my feelings first, surround myself with better people, and keep moving forward.

Techniques for Cultivating a Positive Mindset:

1. Be Kind to Yourself: Treat yourself with compassion. Everyone makes mistakes, what matters is how we move forward.
2. Practice Self-Care: Prioritize your well-being. When you feel overwhelmed, pause and focus on something that brings you joy or comfort, even something as simple as smiling.
3. Focus on Joy and Gratitude: Notice the small, joyful moments in daily life. Gratitude amplifies positivity and abundance. There are some even on the tough days, find one thing to be grateful for.
4. Shift Your Perspective: Use mindfulness, meditation, or breathwork to tune into the present moment. Let go of resistance and focus on what feels right.
5. Align with Your Authentic Self: Act from a place of authenticity. When you live in alignment with your true self, you attract opportunities and relationships that resonate with your values.

Lifespan vs. Healthspan: A Paradigm Shift

In 1919, the average life expectancy in the U.S. was 56 years. Today, it's almost 79. While we've added years to our lifespan, the quality of those years our healthspan is often overlooked.

Healthspan refers to the time we spend in good health, free from chronic disease and physical decline. Extending healthspan, not just lifespan, should be our goal. A healthy life is about more than avoiding disease; it's about complete physical, mental, and social well-being.

The Healthspan-Lifespan Gap

The global population has more than tripled, from 2.9 billion in 1950 to 7.8 billion in 2020. Alongside this growth, life expectancy, a key measure of health has increased from 47 to 73 years. While living longer is a tremendous achievement, the quality of those extra years has become the new focus.

For much of the past century, efforts centered on increasing lifespan, but today, attention is shifting toward expanding healthspan—the years of life spent in good health, free from chronic disease and disability. This shift is especially critical as older populations grow. For example, in the United States, the number of adults over 65 is projected to more than double by 2060, outnumbering children for the first time.

Unfortunately, our healthcare system remains largely focused on treating symptoms and prolonging life rather than preventing disease or addressing root causes. The result is a growing gap between lifespan and healthspan, leaving many people living longer but not healthier lives.

What Is a Healthspan?

Healthspan is more than a single metric; it's a combination of functional measures physical, mental, and emotional that vary from person to person. It's not just about avoiding disease but maintaining vitality and independence throughout life.

To increase healthspan, we must prioritize preventing chronic conditions like cardiovascular disease, diabetes, cancer, and neurodegenerative disorders. Research shows that behaviors such as regular exercise, proper breathing, good nutrition, and a positive mindset can significantly reduce the risk of these conditions, even as we age.

Actionable Steps to Increase Healthspan

1. Move Regularly: Activities like walking, biking, or 30 minutes of exercise a day can lower the risk of chronic diseases such as stroke, diabetes, and high blood pressure.
2. Breathe Properly: Nasal breathing improves oxygen delivery, reduces stress, and supports systemic health, extending both lifespan and healthspan.
3. Cultivate Happiness: A positive mindset and gratitude can improve health outcomes. Studies show that happy people live longer and healthier lives.
4. Prioritize Prevention: Regular checkups and proactive health measures can identify potential issues before symptoms arise.

Take Responsibility for Your Health

Ultimately, you know your body best. While healthcare providers offer guidance, the responsibility for your health lies with you. Becoming informed and proactive allows you to make choices that support long-term wellness rather than temporary fixes.

Our healthcare system excels at treating symptoms but often neglects the root causes. To truly thrive, we must view the body as an interconnected whole. When you listen to your body, meet its needs, and take ownership of your choices, you unlock the potential for a vibrant and fulfilling life.

Call to Action

- Reflect on your health journey. Are you where you want to be?
- Notice how your emotions, habits, and thoughts influence your health.
- Make small, consistent changes that align with your goals.

Remember: your health is your greatest asset. You can't pour from an empty cup. Put yourself first, and everything else will fall into place.

The Evolution of Dental Insurance

Dental care and medical care have historically been treated as separate entities. While medical insurance has existed since 1850, dental insurance only began in 1956 as a benefit negotiated by unions. Today, dental insurance remains limited in scope:

- Coverage amounts have barely increased since the 1950s, often capped at $1,500 annually, which does not reflect inflation or rising costs of care.
- Many people believe that if insurance doesn't cover a procedure, it must not be necessary.

The separation between medical and dental care is counterproductive, as the two are deeply interconnected. This siloed approach has contributed to a health crisis, with cavities being the #1 preventable childhood disease and 70 million Americans suffering from sleep disorders.

A New Approach: Integrating the Mouth and Body

The oral-systemic link underscores how the health of your mouth impacts your overall health. Chronic conditions like anxiety, depression, heart disease, and even cancer can stem from oral health issues. Conversely, habits that support oral health—like proper breathing and regular dental care can enhance systemic health.

The Importance of Early Detection

Diseases like cancer can grow in the body for 5–8 years before symptoms become apparent. Proactive health measures, including attention to oral health, can help detect issues early and prevent invasive interventions. For example, I discovered my breast cancer not through routine tests but by noticing unusual bleeding gums a sign my body was out of balance.

Your body gives you signals; learning to recognize and act on them is key to maintaining both healthspan and lifespan.

Call to Action: Take Charge of Your Healthspan

- Focus on prevention by adopting habits that enhance both oral and overall health.
- Listen to your body and seek care when something feels off.
- Recognize that your thoughts, habits, and mindset are powerful tools in shaping your health and longevity.

As the gap between lifespan and healthspan becomes more apparent, the need for a proactive, whole-body approach to health is clear. By addressing the connections between your mind, mouth, and body, you can not only live longer but live better. Start with small, actionable steps today because your health is the foundation for everything else in life.

When we approach health from a place of positivity and empowerment, we set the stage for success in every aspect of our well-being. This mindset will serve as a cornerstone for the strategies you'll discover in the O.W.N.E.R. framework, helping you breathe better, sleep deeply, and live fully. Let's start by exploring these foundational pillars, beginning with the most vital of all oxygen.

CHAPTER 3

O = Oxygen: Breathing for Life and Wellness

Breathe for Life

We begin and end life with a breath. At birth, our first action is to inhale through our nose. At death, our final action is to exhale, often through our mouth. In between, breath sustains us, delivering the oxygen that fuels every cell, every thought, and every movement.

While we can live weeks without food and days without water, we can only survive **six minutes without oxygen**. Despite its critical importance, most people take breathing for granted, unaware of its profound impact on health, energy, and emotional balance.

This chapter explores why oxygen and proper breathing are the foundations of health, how improper habits can lead to chronic issues, and what you can do today to breathe better, live better, and thrive.

The Science of Breathing

Breathing is a vital function that delivers oxygen to the body and removes carbon dioxide. Oxygen is essential for cellular respiration, the process by which cells convert food into energy. Here's how it works:

1. When you inhale, oxygen enters the lungs and is absorbed into the bloodstream through tiny air sacs called alveoli.
2. Hemoglobin in red blood cells transports oxygen to every cell in the body.
3. At the cellular level, oxygen is combined with glucose to produce adenosine triphosphate (ATP), the energy source for everything from muscle contractions to brain activity.

Why Oxygen Matters

Oxygen fuels nearly every process in the body:

- **Brain Function**: The brain consumes 20% of the body's oxygen. Even a small drop can impair memory, focus, and mood.
- **Cellular Energy**: About 90% of your energy comes from oxygen, with the remaining 10% from food and water.
- **Immune System**: Oxygen helps detoxify cells and fight inflammation.

When oxygen levels are insufficient, the body suffers. Over time, this can lead to fatigue, poor concentration, weakened immunity, and chronic diseases like hypertension, diabetes, and cardiovascular problems.

The Mouth vs. Nose Debate

How you breathe is just as important. Nasal breathing is the body's designed method, offering benefits that mouth breathing cannot match:

1. **Filters Air**: Nose hairs and mucus trap dust, bacteria, and toxins, preventing them from entering the lungs.
2. **Warms and Humidifies**: The nasal passages condition air to the right temperature and humidity for optimal absorption.
3. **Improves Oxygen Efficiency**: Nasal breathing produces nitric oxide, which enhances oxygen uptake and delivery to cells.

In contrast, mouth breathing bypasses these processes, leading to:

- Dry mouth and sore throat.
- Reduced oxygen efficiency.
- Increased risk of gum disease, tooth decay, and systemic inflammation.

Spotting Mouth Breathing

Do you or a loved one experience the following?

- Snoring or disrupted sleep.
- Dry mouth or bad breath upon waking.
- Night sweats or bedwetting (in children).
- Fatigue, brain fog, or irritability during the day.

These symptoms could indicate improper breathing, which often contributes to conditions like Sleep-Disordered Breathing (SDB) or obstructive sleep apnea.

Case Study: My Daughter's Misdiagnosis

When my daughter was young, she experienced night sweats, bedwetting, and behavioral challenges. Doctors suggested ADHD medication, but I suspected something deeper. After years of searching, we discovered she was mouth breathing at night, depriving her brain of oxygen. I am a dental hygienist, her Dad was a dentist and her grandfather an orthodontist none of us were taught to look at tongue function.

Addressing her tongue function and breathing habits transformed her health: the bedwetting stopped, her energy and focus improved, and her behavior stabilized. I had no idea she was in a constant state of fight or flight and was sleep deprived. The brain is the reason for the bedwetting, so it is not a bladder issue. The brain tells the body to get rid of anything you don't need so night sweats and bedwetting are the result. We saw several providers trying everything recommended to stop the bedwetting to no avail until myofunctional therapy. This experience taught me how critical it is to address root causes, not just treat symptoms. How our kids breathe will determine how they grow and develop. Breathing is life. There are so many books on this topic now.

Breathing in Culture and History

For centuries, cultures around the world have recognized the power of breath:

- **Pranayama (India):** Yogic breathing techniques balance energy and calm the mind.
- **Qi Breathing (China):** In traditional Chinese medicine, breath connects the body to life force energy.
- **Catlin's Advocacy (1800s):** George Catlin's book *Shut Your Mouth and Save Your Life* warned of the dangers of mouth breathing, even in the 19th century.

These ancient practices remind us that breathing isn't just a physical act—it's a tool for mental, emotional, and spiritual well-being.

The Domino Effect of Poor Breathing

Improper breathing affects every aspect of health:

- **In Children**: Mouth breathing can lead to developmental issues like elongated facial structure, narrow palates, and crowded teeth.
- **In Adults**: Chronic mouth breathing contributes to fatigue, anxiety, and systemic inflammation.
- **In Overall Health**: Reduced oxygen impacts cellular energy, immune response, and brain function.

Practical Step for Better Breathing

1. **Perform a Breathing Self-Check**
   - Observe how often your mouth is open during the day.
   - Notice whether you wake up with a dry mouth or snore at night.
2. **Practice Nasal Hygiene**
   - Use a warm washcloth or nasal rinse like Xlear ™ to clear your nasal passages daily.
3. **Incorporate Breathing Exercises**.

How to Perform a Breathing Self-Check

Ensuring you can breathe effectively through both nostrils is a simple yet essential test for nasal health. Here's how you can perform a quick self-check:

1. Nostril Test:
   - Gently press one nostril closed with your finger and breathe in through the open nostril.
   - Repeat this process on the other side.
   - Pay attention to whether you can breathe easily through both nostrils. If one side feels significantly more blocked, it may indicate congestion or other nasal issues.
2. Hold-and-Breathe Test:
   - Hold both nostrils closed with your fingers for a moment.
   - Release your grip and try to breathe through your nose without opening your mouth.

- Notice if you can comfortably draw air in through your nostrils. Difficulty in breathing this way might suggest partial or complete nasal blockage.
3. Condensation Test with Your Phone:
   - Take your phone and make the screen black (turn off the display or use a dark background).
   - Hold the phone close to your nose and exhale onto the screen.
   - Look at the condensation pattern left behind. Do you see an equal amount of condensation from both nostrils?
   - Unequal patterns or a lack of condensation on one side might suggest restricted airflow in that nostril.

This simple self-check can help you assess if there's any imbalance in your nasal breathing. If you notice persistent issues, it may be time to incorporate nasal hygiene into your routine or consult a healthcare professional.

Nasal Hygiene

Your nose is essential for conditioning the air you breathe and for maintaining a disease-free body.

From a very young age, we learn the importance of dental hygiene. As critical as dental health is for our well-being, the same goes for nasal health. Most often, we tend to ignore it, and there is a lack of awareness about its importance. However, since the Covid-19 pandemic and the new habits formed from prolonged mask-wearing, people across the globe are viewing nasal hygiene through a different lens and becoming increasingly aware of its importance.

Why is nasal hygiene so important?

Your nose plays a critical role in conditioning the air you breathe by humidifying, warming, and filtering it. These functions ensure that the air is optimized for oxygen exchange in your lungs while also protecting you from environmental pollutants, bacteria, viruses, and other particulates.

Since your nostrils are directly exposed to environmental air, they can accumulate dust, pollution, bacteria, and fungi. These foreign substances can trigger infections and illnesses. By maintaining good nasal hygiene, you can improve the quality of the air entering your lungs and reduce your risk of illness, congestion, and discomfort.

Practicing proper nasal hygiene not only supports your nose's natural functions but can also provide additional health benefits. You may find it easier to breathe, feel more energetic, and notice an improvement in your overall quality of life.

True Nasal Hygiene

True nasal hygiene involves keeping your nasal passages clean, clear, and moisturized to ensure your nose functions at peak performance. Rather than waiting for symptoms to appear, you can proactively rinse away dust, allergens, and other irritants from your sinuses.

Proper nasal hygiene can:

- Relieve allergy symptoms.
- Reduce the chances of an asthma attack.
- Enhance your ability to breathe comfortably and feel better overall.
- Shorten the duration and intensity of illnesses.

By taking just a few minutes a day to care for your nasal passages, you may also experience clearer thinking, improved focus, and increased energy levels.

Causes and Remedies for Dry Nasal Passages

Dry nasal passages can result from various factors, including:

- Colds or allergies.
- Mouth breathing.
- Overuse of antihistamines or decongestants.
- Exposure to smoke or poor air quality.
- Weather changes, air conditioning, or heating.
- Certain medications or surgeries.

When nasal passages become dry, symptoms such as irritation, burning, or inflammation may occur. Addressing the root cause is key, but you can often find relief with:

- Nasal-safe moisturizing drops or rinses (e.g., Xlear).
- Using a humidifier.
- Steam treatments.
- Staying hydrated.

For severe cases, it's important to:

- Stop overusing OTC nasal sprays and medications.
- Consult a healthcare professional to determine the underlying cause.

Incorporating Nasal Care Into Your Routine

Many people ask about the best time to clean their noses. I recommend rinsing your nasal passages once in the morning to remove pollutants accumulated overnight and once in the evening to clear out debris from the day. For infants, using saline drops (like Xlear) during diaper changes can help keep their nasal passages stay clear and moisturized.

By simply adding nasal care to your daily routine, you can reduce the frequency and severity of illnesses, improve your breathing, and reclaim a sense of clarity and control over your life.

Nose-Unblocking Exercise

If your nose feels congested, and nasal hygiene does not work to clear it, you can try this simple exercise to help open your nasal passages naturally:

1. **Prepare Yourself:**
    - Sit upright in a comfortable position and take a few normal breaths through your nose if possible. If your nose is completely blocked, breathe gently through your mouth to start.
2. **Controlled Breathing:**
    - Take a small, gentle breath in through your nose (or mouth if necessary).
    - Exhale softly and completely through your nose.

3. **Hold Your Breath:**
   - After exhaling, pinch your nostrils shut with your fingers to block your nose completely.
   - Keep your mouth closed and hold your breath.
4. **Head Movements:**
   - While holding your breath, nod your head up and down or gently sway your upper body side to side to distract yourself and increase CO_2 buildup.
5. **Release and Breathe:**
   - When you feel a strong urge to breathe, let go of your nose and breathe in gently through your nostrils.
   - Avoid gasping; instead, try to maintain calm, controlled breathing.
6. **Repeat as Needed:**
   - Wait about 30 seconds, then repeat the process up to 5 times. You should notice your nasal passages becoming clearer.

Why Does This Work?

This exercise increases carbon dioxide levels in your body, which can help dilate the nasal passages and relieve congestion. It's a simple and natural way to improve airflow without relying on medications or sprays.

Tip: After unblocking your nose, rinse your nasal passages with a saline solution or nasal spray to remove mucus and allergens to maintain clarity.

Breathing Exercises for Health

1. **Diaphragmatic (Belly) Breathing**
   - Sit or lie comfortably. Place one hand on your chest and one on your belly.
   - Inhale deeply through your nose, expanding your belly. Keep your chest still.
   - Exhale slowly through your nose, letting your belly fall naturally.
2. **Box Breathing (4-4-4-4)**
   - Inhale through your nose for 4 seconds.

- Hold your breath for 4 seconds.
- Exhale through your nose for 4 seconds.
- Pause for 4 seconds before repeating.

3. **Alternate Nostril Breathing (Nadi Shodhana)**
   - Close one nostril, inhale through the other. Switch and exhale through the opposite nostril.

4. **4-7-8 Breathing**
   - Inhale for 4 seconds, hold for 7 seconds, and exhale for 8 seconds.

Connecting Breath to Other Principles

Oxygen is the first building block of health, but it doesn't work alone. Proper breathing:

- Enhances hydration by improving blood flow (Water).
- Supports cellular metabolism, powered by nutrients (Nutrition).
- Improves sleep quality, essential for recovery (Sleep).
- Encourages respect for your body's natural rhythms and needs (Respect).

When to Seek Professional Help

If you find that you consistently cannot breathe through your nose despite trying nasal hygiene practices and exercises, it's important to consult a healthcare professional. Persistent nasal blockage or difficulty breathing through your nose could indicate underlying issues such as:

- Structural problems (e.g., a deviated septum or nasal polyps).
- Chronic sinusitis or nasal infections.
- Severe allergies.
- Non-allergic rhinitis or inflammation.
- Enlarged adenoids or other anatomical abnormalities.

An **Ear, Nose, and Throat (ENT) specialist** is trained to evaluate and treat conditions affecting the nasal passages and sinuses. They may perform a thorough examination, recommend imaging studies, or suggest treatments ranging from medications to surgical interventions, depending on the cause of your nasal obstruction.

Don't delay seeking help if:

- You experience persistent congestion that doesn't improve with nasal hygiene routines or over-the-counter remedies.
- You notice recurring headaches, facial pain, or pressure.
- You struggle to sleep due to nasal blockage or mouth breathing.
- Your ability to smell or taste is significantly impaired.

Addressing the root cause of your nasal breathing difficulties can help restore proper airflow, improve oxygen intake, and enhance your overall quality of life.

Call to Action

B.R.E.A.T.H.E. Better System

Focus: Breathing is the simplest, most accessible tool you have for improving your health. Start with these steps:

Key Steps:

- **B**reathe: Teach proper nasal breathing techniques.
- **R**elax: Incorporate stress management practices like mindful breathing.
- **E**valuate: Observe your breathing habits and nasal hygiene
- **A**djust: Correct improper breathing and tongue posture through simple exercises.
- **T**rain: Practice daily breathing and myofunctional exercises for long-term results.
- **H**ydrate: Stay hydrated to support breathing and airway health.
- **E**levate: Create consistent habits to optimize energy and well-being.

Remember, every breath is a chance to reset your body and mind. By focusing on this fundamental principle, you lay the foundation for a longer, healthier, and more vibrant life.

While oxygen fuels every cell, it cannot work alone. Water is its essential partner, ensuring delivery and balance within the body. Breathing provides the oxygen your body needs to survive, but oxygen alone can't do its job without water. Oxygen relies on water to transport it through your bloodstream, power cellular processes, and keep your organs functioning.

Just as dehydration can impair oxygen delivery, improper hydration throws your entire system out of balance. Water isn't just a companion to oxygen—it's the next essential pillar of health.

CHAPTER 4

W = Water: Hydration for Health

Water: More Than Just Hydration

Water, like oxygen, is essential for life. Without oxygen, survival is measured in minutes; without water, it's a matter of days. Yet water is far more than just a survival tool, it is the foundation for physical and mental vitality. It powers cellular functions, supports digestion, regulates temperature, and even aids the delivery of oxygen to every cell in your body.

Despite water's importance, a staggering 75% of people are chronically dehydrated, putting them at risk for fatigue, brain fog, and long-term health issues. Beyond just drinking enough, ensuring the quality of your water is equally critical.

Water is the second pillar of health because it builds on oxygen to sustain every system in the body. Let's dive into why water is essential, how much you need, and how to ensure it's clean and nourishing.

Why Water Is Essential to Life

Water plays a vital role in your body's daily functions:

1. **Cellular Support**: Water delivers oxygen and nutrients to cells, removes waste, and keeps tissues hydrated.
2. **Detoxification**: Kidneys and the liver use water to flush out toxins. Without enough water, these organs struggle to function effectively.
3. **Temperature Regulation**: Sweating cools the body and prevents overheating, especially in hot climates or during exercise.
4. **Joint Lubrication**: Water cushions joints, reducing friction and discomfort during movement.
5. **Digestion**: From saliva production to the absorption of nutrients, water is essential for a healthy digestive system.

Without sufficient hydration, these systems begin to break down, leading to immediate and long-term health challenges.

How much water should you drink a day? Like most things in life there is no one size fits all answer. Most people need about four to six cups of plain water each day for generally healthy people, that amount differs based on how much water they take in from other beverages and food sources. Also, certain health conditions, medications, activity level, and ambient temperature influence total daily water intake. If you don't drink enough water each day, you risk becoming dehydrated.

Unfortunately, many of us aren't getting enough to drink, especially older adults. We'll help you understand how much water you need to drink in a day to stay healthy.

Water keeps every system in the body functioning properly. The Harvard Medical School Reports that water has many important jobs, such as:

- carrying nutrients and oxygen to your cells
- flushing bacteria from your bladder
- aiding digestion
- preventing constipation
- normalizing blood pressure
- cushioning joints
- protecting organs and tissues
- regulating body temperature
- maintaining electrolyte (sodium) balance.

When considering the water in your body, think about this: While it's true that we are primarily made up of water, none of it is plain $H2O$. For your drink to be easily absorbed within the gut and to spread into the cells that need it most, it needs to have the right mix of water and electrolytes.

To get the correct mix of water and electrolytes, you can either drink naturally electrolyte-rich beverages like coconut water, or add a small pinch of salt (like sea salt) to your regular water. Most people know salt contains sodium, but it actually also contains the minerals potassium, calcium, and magnesium. Sea salt and Himalayan pink salt are the best types of salt to add to water as they are less processed than normal table salt.

For more intense exercise, consider a commercially prepared sports drink with a balanced electrolyte profile, or you can purchase electrolyte packets to add to your water. Always consult your doctor if you have concerns about electrolyte balance or water intake.

How to Make Electrolyte Water for Dehydration

- Water: Start with 4 cups of water.
- Salt (optional): Get 1/4 to 1/2 teaspoon of salt.
- Sugar or Sweetener: Use 2-4 tablespoons of a sweetener of your choice, such as honey, agave nectar, or sugar.
- Potassium chloride powder.
- Magnesium malate powder.
- Citrus Juice: Add juice from half a lemon or half an orange.

The Importance of Water Quality: Our Family Story

Understanding the importance of clean water hits close to home for me. My mother-in-law, who never smoked a day in her life, was diagnosed with lung cancer. For years, she lived on the banks of the Kankakee River, which has long been known for pollution from agricultural runoff, industrial waste, and other contaminants.

While we may never know for sure, she always believed her cancer was tied to the water she drank that the city took from the river. It was her only water source for years before advanced filtration systems were available. She would often say, "You can't see what's in the water, it's not safe. We often worry about water shortages in third-world countries, but have we stopped to consider the quality of our own water supply?"

Her story is a heartbreaking reminder that water is more than just hydration, it can carry invisible dangers that affect your health over time. It's why I'm so passionate about educating others on the importance of not just drinking water, but ensuring it's clean and free from harmful contaminants. That's why I urge everyone to take a closer look at their water supply. Something as simple as installing a filter can be life-changing.

How to Ensure Safe, Clean Water

You don't need to be a water expert to protect yourself and your family. For those with access to water, taking a few simple steps can dramatically improve your water quality:

Step 1: Test Your Water

- Start with a home water testing kit to detect contaminants like lead, nitrates, or bacteria.
- If you're not sure where to begin, consider reaching out to your local water provider for an annual water quality report.

Step 2: Choose the Right Source

- Tap water may require filtering for safety.
- Bottled water often contains microplastics and isn't always better than filtered tap water.
- Spring water is mineral-rich but should be tested for contaminants.

Step 3: Filter Your Water

Different filters address different concerns, so it's important to match your filter to your water's needs:

- **For Chlorine and Odors**: Activated carbon filters, like those in Brita or PUR pitchers, are affordable and effective for basic filtration.
- **For Heavy Metals or Fluoride**: Reverse osmosis systems, such as AquaTru, are ideal for removing lead, arsenic, and fluoride.
- **For Bacteria and Emergencies**: Portable options like LifeStraw filters are great for travel, camping, or emergency preparedness.
- **For Whole-House Solutions**: Systems like Culligan provide comprehensive filtration for both drinking and bathing water.

Step 3: Where to Get Safe and Clean Water Consider Advanced Options

Ensuring access to clean water doesn't have to be complicated. There are many reliable brands and systems available to meet different needs, whether you're filtering water at home, on the go, or for emergency preparedness.

For those who want to go beyond basic filtration here are some trusted options:

1. **Berkey Water Filters**
   - What It Does: Known for gravity-fed water filtration systems, Berkey removes heavy metals, bacteria, viruses, pesticides, and other harmful contaminants.
   - Why It's Great:
     o Portable and ideal for home use or emergency preparedness.
     o No electricity or plumbing required.
     o Long-lasting filters with high capacity.

2. **Kangen Water Machines**
   - What It Does: Kangen machines produce alkaline, ionized water by filtering and then electrolyzing tap water.
   - Why It's Great:
     o Produces water with a higher pH, which some believe helps balance body acidity.
     o Multi-use: Provides water for drinking, cooking, cleaning, and skincare.
     o Compact and suitable for countertop use.

3. **Hydroviv Custom Water Filters**
   - What It Does: Hydroviv specializes in creating water filters tailored to your local water supply. By analyzing the specific contaminants in your area, their filters are designed to target issues like lead, arsenic, PFAS (forever chemicals), and chlorine.
   - Why It's Great:
     o Customized to address your specific water quality concerns.
     o Ideal for regions with known contamination issues or aging infrastructure.
     o Easy to install and use, with options for under-sink systems.

4. **Culligan Water Systems**
   - What It Does: Culligan specializes in whole-house filtration systems, water softeners, and **(RO) Reverse Osmosis Systems**: Eliminate heavy metals and fluoride
   - Why It's Great:

- Customizable systems to target specific contaminants in your local water supply.
- Professional installation and maintenance.
- Great for families or anyone looking to improve both drinking and bathing water quality.

5. **Brita and PUR Filters**
- What They Do: Affordable pitcher and faucet filters that remove basic contaminants like chlorine, lead, and sediment.
- Why They're Great:
  - Budget-friendly and widely available.
  - Easy to use and maintain.
  - A good starting option for light filtration needs.

6. **AquaTru Reverse Osmosis**
- What It Does: Countertop reverse osmosis (RO) system that removes hundreds of contaminants, including fluoride, arsenic, and heavy metals.
- Why It's Great:
  - Compact design for kitchens.
  - Removes up to 99% of impurities.
  - No plumbing required, making it easy to set up and use.

7. **LifeStraw Personal and Family Filters**
- What It Does: Portable water purification devices that remove bacteria, parasites, and microplastics.
- Why It's Great:
  - Ideal for camping, travel, or emergency use.
  - Lightweight and easy to carry.
  - Affordable and effective in survival situations.

8. **Local Water Delivery Services**
- Many companies, like Primo Water or Crystal Springs, deliver purified or spring water in large reusable containers.
- Why It's Great:
- Convenient and eco-friendly.

- Perfect for homes, offices, or those who prefer a refillable option.

How to Choose the Right Water Solution

1. Assess Your Needs:
   - For everyday home use: Consider systems like Berkey, Culligan, or AquaTru.
   - For travel or emergencies: Portable options like LifeStraw or Berkey Go make sense.
   - For health-conscious consumers: Kangen or AquaTru may align with your goals.
2. Test Your Water:
   - Use a home water testing kit to determine what contaminants are in your supply.
3. Research Local Resources:
   - Check if your area offers refillable water stations or community filtration systems.
4. Factor in Convenience:
   - If you're on a budget, start with affordable solutions like Brita or PUR.
   - For long-term or whole-house needs, invest in professional systems like Culligan.

Optimize Hydration

- Start your day with a glass of water to rehydrate after sleep.
- Add lemon or baking soda to water for a pH boost.
- Incorporate water-rich foods like cucumbers and watermelon.

Global Challenges to Clean Water

While many of us have access to clean water, billions face shortages or contamination:

- **2 Billion Without Safe Water**: According to the WHO, 1 in 4 people lack access to clean drinking water.
- **Climate Change**: Droughts and flooding exacerbate water scarcity and contamination.

- **Waterborne Diseases**: Contaminated water leads to illnesses like cholera and typhoid, disproportionately affecting children.

Clean water is not just a personal health issue, it's a global crisis.

Connecting Water to Other Health Principles

Water is essential, but it doesn't work alone. It complements the other pillars of health:

- **Oxygen**: Water transports oxygen to cells, making hydration critical for energy.
- **Nutrition**: Water aids digestion and nutrient absorption, ensuring your body gets the fuel it needs.
- **Sleep**: Dehydration disrupts sleep, impacting recovery and repair.

Water: The Foundation for Vitality

Water lays the groundwork for health by hydrating your cells, supporting oxygen delivery, and maintaining balance throughout your body. But hydration alone isn't enough. For true vitality, your body also needs the right nutrients, the essential building blocks that fuel energy, growth, and repair.

Just as the quality of your water impacts every part of your health, so does the food you consume. Nutrition, the third pillar of health, takes hydration to the next level by providing the energy your body needs to function at its best. Together, hydration and nutrition create the foundation for a vibrant, thriving body.

Call to Action

Hydration isn't just about survival, it's about thriving. By drinking enough clean, high-quality water, you give your body the tools it needs to perform at its best. Take the first step today:

- Grab a glass of water.
- Test your water supply.
- Make hydration a part of your daily routine.

This was one of the hardest parts of my healing journey to figure out. What system to use, what water was best. If you are confused about where to start please reach out.

Hydration and Its Impact on Systemic Health

To help you visualize the profound difference hydration makes in your body, let's compare the effectiveness of key health aspects when the body is hydrated versus dehydrated:

Health Aspect	Effectiveness When Hydrated	Effectiveness When Dehydrated
Energy Levels	90%	50%
Brain Function	85%	45%
Detoxification	80%	40%
Digestion	85%	50%
Joint Health	80%	40%

Key Takeaways:

- **Hydration powers your body.** From energy levels to digestion and detoxification, proper hydration allows your body to function at its best.

- **Dehydration impacts everything.** Even mild dehydration can reduce effectiveness in crucial systems by nearly half.

Why This Matters

Hydration is more than just quenching thirst, it's the foundation for your body's ability to perform, repair, and heal. By making hydration a daily priority, you can unlock peak performance in both your physical and mental health.

In the next chapter, we'll explore the third pillar of health: nutrition. You'll learn how the food you eat fuels your body, shapes your mind, impacts your future and the vital connection between what you eat and how you feel.

CHAPTER 5

N = Nutrition: Food as Medicine and Nourishment

Nourish to Flourish—Food Is Medicine

After addressing the vital roles of oxygen and water, it's time to focus on the third pillar of health: nutrition. While oxygen and water sustain your body at the most basic level, nutrition fuels every process from cellular repair to brain function. Without proper nutrition, even the benefits of hydration and oxygen delivery fall short, leaving your body underpowered and vulnerable.

The old saying, "You are what you eat," couldn't be more true. Food has the power to heal or harm. It can energize us or cause inflammation, leaving us susceptible to chronic diseases. Over time, our understanding of nutrition has evolved from ancestral diets to the heavily processed foods lining our grocery store shelves today. To truly nourish our bodies, we must understand the profound impact food has on our health.

The Evolution of Food: From Nature to Additives

Before the agricultural revolution, food came directly from nature. Early humans consumed a diet rich in variety, fruits, vegetables, nuts, seeds, and lean meats from wild game. These foods were nutrient-dense, free from chemicals, and in harmony with what the body needed.

The agricultural revolution, roughly 10,000 years ago, marked a turning point in human diets. Grains became a staple, and farming allowed for more consistent food production. While this shift brought population growth and stability, it also introduced challenges. Diets became more carbohydrate-heavy, and the diversity of nutrients began to decline. Over centuries, the rise of industrial farming further shifted the focus from quality to quantity. Modern farming practices, focused on maximizing yield, stripped the soil of its nutrients, leaving crops less nutritious than their ancestral counterparts.

Today, we face an abundance of processed foods laden with additives, preservatives, and artificial flavors. These foods may be convenient, but they are often low in essential nutrients and high in sugars, unhealthy fats, and chemicals. As Gary Brecka, a longevity expert, points out, "The more steps food takes to reach your plate, the less life it brings to your body."

The Role of Nutrition in Your Body

Every bite of food you eat sends instructions to your body. These instructions can be healing or harmful. Proper nutrition supports cellular repair, balances hormones, boosts the immune system, and fuels brain function. On the other hand, nutrient deficiencies and inflammatory foods disrupt these processes, leading to fatigue, disease, and mental fog.

Dr. Livingood, a natural health advocate, stresses that chronic inflammation often driven by diet is the root cause of many modern illnesses. Foods high in added sugars, refined grains, and unhealthy fats can trigger this inflammation, while whole, nutrient-dense foods can calm it. The gut, often called the "second brain," plays a central role in this process.

When you fuel your body with processed or inflammatory foods, it's like putting cheap, low-grade oil into a finely tuned machine—it might keep running for a while, but over time, the wear and tear start to show. These foods are often stripped of nutrients and loaded with additives, preservatives, and unhealthy fats that can disrupt your body's natural balance. Instead of providing energy, they can leave you feeling sluggish, bloated, and inflamed. Over time, this constant internal stress can lead to chronic conditions, fatigue, and even a weakened immune system. Your body craves whole, nourishing foods that work with it, not against it, to thrive and repair. When we eat poorly, our body whispers through discomfort, and if ignored, it begins to shout through disease.

The Power of Food to Heal or Harm

Every meal you eat sends instructions to your body. These instructions can either promote healing or cause harm. Foods rich in nutrients provide your body with the building blocks it needs for energy, repair, and resilience. On the other hand, foods high in sugar, unhealthy fats, and artificial additives contribute to inflammation, insulin resistance, and other chronic conditions.

For example:

- **Healing Foods:**
  - Leafy greens like spinach and kale are packed with vitamins, minerals, and antioxidants that fight inflammation.
  - Fermented foods like yogurt and sauerkraut support gut health and improve digestion.
  - Healthy fats from avocados, nuts, and seeds provide long-lasting energy and support brain function.
- **Harmful Foods:**
  - Sugary drinks and snacks cause blood sugar spikes and crashes, leading to fatigue and weight gain.
  - Processed meats and fried foods are high in trans fats, which increase inflammation and cardiovascular risk.
  - Artificial additives and preservatives can disrupt the gut microbiome and burden the liver.

Food as Medicine: The Foundation of Wellness and The Role of Gut Health:

Your gut is home to trillions of microorganisms that form your microbiome. This microbiome plays a central role in digestion, immunity, and even mental health. When the gut is balanced, it supports everything from nutrient absorption to mood regulation. It sends signals of wellness to the brain, resulting in mental clarity, emotional stability, and a sense of balance. However, when it's disrupted by poor nutrition, stress, or antibiotics, the entire body can suffer. A diet rich in prebiotic and probiotic foods, like leafy greens, fermented vegetables, and yogurt, can nurture a healthy gut microbiome, setting the stage for better overall health.

A gut-friendly diet includes:

- **Probiotics:** Found in fermented foods like kefir, kimchi, and miso, these beneficial bacteria restore gut balance.
- **Prebiotics:** Fiber-rich foods like onions, garlic, and bananas feed the good bacteria in your gut.

- **Anti-Inflammatory Foods:** Turmeric, ginger, and green tea calm inflammation in the gut lining.

When your gut is healthy, it sends signals to your brain that promote mental clarity, emotional stability, and overall well-being. This gut-brain connection is a powerful reminder that what you eat affects how you think and feel.

Nutrition doesn't just affect you it can influence future generations. Epigenetics, as mentioned earlier is the study of how behaviors and environment influence gene expression, has shown that your diet can "turn on" or "turn off" certain genes.

For example, eating antioxidant-rich foods can protect your DNA from damage, while a diet high in processed foods can activate genes linked to inflammation and disease. These changes aren't permanent; you have the power to reverse harmful patterns by making healthier choices.

The Invisible Battle: Understanding Oxidative Stress

Have you ever wondered why some people seem to age faster, feel more fatigued, or are more prone to illness, even when they seem relatively healthy? The answer often lies in an invisible battle happening inside their bodies, one driven by oxidative stress.

Oxidative stress occurs when there's an imbalance between free radicals and antioxidants in the body. Free radicals are unstable molecules missing an electron, and they act like reckless burglars, scavenging your body and "stealing" electrons from healthy cells. This creates a cascade of damage that can harm your cells, proteins, and even your DNA. Over time, this process accelerates aging and lays the groundwork for chronic diseases like heart disease, diabetes, and even cancer. This is why the basics oxygen, water, nutrition and sleep need to be a priority.

Why Oxidative Stress Matters

This cellular damage doesn't just affect how you feel it impacts how you function.

- **Aging:** Oxidative stress speeds up visible signs of aging, such as wrinkles and skin sagging, while also weakening your internal systems.

- **Chronic Disease:** Free radicals can damage blood vessels, contributing to conditions like high blood pressure and atherosclerosis, which increase the risk of heart attacks and strokes.
- **Oral Health:** In your mouth, oxidative stress contributes to gum disease, tooth loss, and even the breakdown of oral tissues, which can trigger inflammation throughout your body.

The good news? You have a natural defense system: antioxidants.

Antioxidants: Your Body's Built-In Defense

Antioxidants are like the superheroes of your body's health, neutralizing free radicals and preventing them from wreaking havoc. They do this by donating an electron to free radicals, stabilizing them without becoming unstable themselves.

Where do these health-boosting superheroes come from? They're in the foods you eat. The key is to include antioxidant-rich choices in your diet daily.

Here are some of the best sources:

- **Berries:** Blueberries, raspberries, and strawberries are loaded with anthocyanins, which protect your brain, heart, and immune system.
- **Green Tea:** Rich in catechins, green tea is a powerful anti-inflammatory and heart-healthy beverage.
- **Leafy Greens:** Spinach and kale contain lutein and zeaxanthin, which support eye and skin health while reducing oxidative stress.
- **Nuts and Seeds:** Almonds, walnuts, and flaxseeds are packed with vitamin E, an antioxidant that helps repair damaged cells.
- **Dark Chocolate:** High-quality dark chocolate (70% cacao or more) is full of flavonoids that promote heart health and boost mood.
- **Colorful Vegetables:** Brightly colored produce like carrots, bell peppers, and tomatoes are rich in carotenoids, which protect against cell damage.

Practical Ways to Fight Oxidative Stress

The best way to combat oxidative stress is to make small, consistent changes in your daily habits. Here's how:

1. **Eat a Rainbow:** Fill your plate with a variety of colorful fruits and vegetables to get a wide range of antioxidants.
2. **Swap Sodas for Green Tea:** A simple change like replacing sugary drinks with antioxidant-rich green tea can make a big impact.
3. **Snack Smart:** Choose nuts, seeds, or dark chocolate instead of processed snacks.
4. **Limit Toxins:** Avoid smoking, excessive alcohol, and processed foods, which can increase oxidative stress.
5. **Embrace Moderate Exercise:** Regular exercise boosts your body's production of natural antioxidants, but avoid overtraining, which can have the opposite effect.
6. **Manage Stress:** Chronic stress increases free radical production, so prioritize relaxation techniques like yoga, deep breathing, or journaling.

Connecting Oxidative Stress to Oral Health

What happens in your mouth doesn't stay in your mouth. Gum disease, for instance, creates a localized environment of oxidative stress that can spill over into your bloodstream, triggering inflammation throughout your body. By reducing oxidative stress with a healthy diet and good oral hygiene, you're protecting more than just your smile you're safeguarding your overall health.

Takeaway Message

Oxidative stress may be an invisible threat, but it's one you can control. With every bite you take, every breath you take, by slowing down, get enough sleep and make every effort to nurture your body to strengthen its natural defenses. By choosing antioxidant-rich foods and balancing your lifestyle, you're giving your body the tools it needs to thrive, today and for years to come.

Overcoming Common Barriers

Let's address some of the most common excuses for not eating healthier:

- **"Healthy food is too expensive."**
  While organic produce and specialty items can be costly, many healthy staples are affordable. Beans, rice, oats, and seasonal vegetables are nutrient-dense and budget-friendly.
- **"I don't have time to cook."**
  Meal prep doesn't have to be complicated. Cook large batches of grains, roast a tray of vegetables, and prep protein sources like chicken or tofu for easy assembly during the week.
- **"I don't know what to eat."**
  Start simple: focus on whole, minimally processed foods. If it comes from the earth or has a short ingredient list, it's likely a good choice.

Bridging the Gap: Knowing vs. Doing

Why do so many of us struggle to make healthy choices, even when we know better? The answer lies in our habits, environment, and mindset. Food is more than fuel; it's comfort, culture, and convenience. Overcoming the pull of unhealthy choices requires conscious effort and practical strategies. There is so much information available on this one subject alone. We all have different likes and dislikes, find what resonates with you and give it a try. It's not rocket science! If what you are doing does not feel right to your body try something else.

The Urgency of Finding Your Optimal Diet

The food you eat provides the building blocks for your body to function. Poor nutrition contributes to fatigue, mental fog, and chronic disease. Finding a diet that works for your unique needs isn't just about health, it's about living your best life.

Take charge of your nutrition today:

- Experiment with foods that energize you and eliminate those that don't.
- Seek support from a nutritionist or trusted resource.
- Commit to small, consistent changes that build over time.

Epigenetics and Nutrition

For decades, we believed our genes dictated our health. While genetics do play a role, epigenetics the study of how behaviors and environment influence gene expression has shown that our choices are far more powerful than we once thought.

Your diet, habits, and even stress levels can turn genes "on" or "off," influencing everything from inflammation to disease risk. This means that what you eat today doesn't just affect you it can impact future generations. Poor nutrition can leave epigenetic markers that predispose your children and grandchildren to health challenges. Conversely, adopting healthy habits can create positive changes that last for generations.

Modern Diets: A Double-Edged Sword

The diet and nutrition industry is booming, yet so many of us are less healthy than ever. In 2022, the global human nutrition market was valued at $383.4 billion, projected to reach $719.69 billion by 2032. Despite this, our diets are often filled with ultra-processed foods that our bodies aren't designed to handle.

Our ancestors didn't face the challenges we do today. They didn't have to decipher food labels filled with unpronounceable chemicals. Their food came from the earth, whole, unprocessed, and nutrient-dense. Compare that to now, where the average person consumes artificial additives, preservatives, and sugars daily. These substances confuse our bodies, leading to inflammation, poor nutrient absorption, and metabolic imbalances.

Even foods we consider healthy, like fruits and vegetables, have lost nutrient density due to industrial farming practices. This is why many people, including health advocates like Gary Brecka, emphasize the importance of supplementation to fill in nutritional gaps.

Personalizing Your Nutrition Plan

Every person's body is unique, which means there is no one-size-fits-all diet. What works for one person may not work for another. Trial and error is often necessary to determine which foods best support your body.

Start by paying attention to how food makes you feel. Keep a journal of what you eat and note changes in energy, mood, or digestion. For example, you might notice fatigue after eating processed carbs or improved focus after a meal rich in healthy fats and vegetables.

For families, teaching children about nutrition is crucial. I've seen firsthand, both in my personal life and professional career, how food choices impact oral and overall health. The bacteria in your mouth, often influenced by diet, doesn't just affect your teeth, it can travel to your gut and bloodstream, influencing systemic health.

Trial and error is the best way to test and see what your kids will eat. When their tongue does not function properly it will cause them to have food aversions. I would yell at my daughter when she spit food out. I thought she was being bad but she had sensory issues with textures. My sister was constantly telling her daughter to chew with her mouth closed.

I now know how the tongue functions plays a big role with picky and noisy eaters. With some kids, their tongue is protecting their airway, keeping them in fight or flight and they cannot chew, swallow and breathe at the same time. That is why they smack their food and chew with their mouth open.

Looking at how the tongue functions is where to start if you are having difficulty with feeding. Go to the tongue chapter and myofunctional therapy for more information on this.

A smoothie is a great way to incorporate the protein and vitamins needed and you can make it taste great especially for picky eaters.

There are many people in the nutrition space that are working to get us back on track. A good rule is if it comes from the earth it is probably good for you.

There are also so many supplements due to the fact that we are not giving our body the nutrients it needs. I have found many plant based supplements I go to when I know I am out of balance. One of my favorite companies is Aroga Life. They have supplements for every system of the body. Another is Asea. There are so many to choose from. These work for me. If you follow a functional medicine doctor they will use the brand they find works for them.

The Urgency of Finding Your Optimal Diet

The food we eat provides the building blocks for all body functions, proper nutrition is a foundation for health, energy, and disease prevention. The urgency of finding the correct diet tailored to your individual needs is high because it directly impacts day-to-day vitality, mental clarity, immune resilience, and long-term health. A balanced, personalized diet allows your body to perform at its best, helping prevent chronic diseases, supporting a healthy weight, and enabling you to age gracefully. Starting now gives you an immediate boost and sets you up for lifelong health.

Action Steps: Take Charge of Your Nutrition

Take Charge of Your Health: Start Your Journey to Proper Nutrition Today! There are so many opinions when it comes to diet and nutrition.

Your body deserves the best fuel to thrive, and the right nutrition is key to unlocking your full potential. Here's how you can start:

1. **Choose Whole Foods:** Whenever possible, opt for foods in their natural state. If it comes from the earth or has minimal processing, it's likely good for you.
2. **Set Small, Achievable Goals:** Begin by making one simple change: swap sugary drinks for water, add a serving of veggies to each meal, or prioritize whole foods over processed options.
3. **Limit Inflammatory Foods:** Reduce your intake of added sugars, refined grains, and artificial additives.
4. **Listen to Your Body:** Pay attention to how different foods make you feel. Notice your energy, mood, and focus. Your body gives clear signals when it's getting the nutrients it needs! Keep a food journal to keep track of how you feel. Experiment and adapt.
5. **Supplement Wisely:** Test to see what your body needs. Consider plant-based supplements like those from Aroga Life or Asea to fill nutritional gaps.
6. **Seek Support:** Consult a nutritionist, join a wellness group, or find a friend who shares your goals. Guidance and accountability can make the journey smoother and more effective.

7. **Commit to Consistency:** True change happens over time. Make nutrition a priority every day, and celebrate the progress you make along the way!
8. **Focus on Education:** Teach your family about the importance of nutrition. Habits formed early in life often last a lifetime.

Food Is Medicine

The food you eat provides the foundation for your health. It has the power to heal, energize, and protect you or to harm and inflame. By making conscious choices and listening to your body's needs, you can unlock a level of vitality and clarity you may never have thought possible.

As we move forward in this journey of health, remember: your choices today don't just affect you. They shape the health of generations to come. Listen to your body, respect its needs, and nourish it with intention.

Your health is worth the effort. You are worth it!

The nutrients you consume provide the building blocks for energy, recovery, and growth but there's one element that amplifies their effectiveness: sleep. Without sufficient sleep, your body can't properly repair tissues, regulate hormones, or process nutrients efficiently.

As we wrap up nutrition, it's important to recognize that fueling your body with the right nutrients is just one piece of the puzzle. While what you eat provides the building blocks for health, your body needs time to process, repair, and restore, this is where the fourth pillar, enough sleep, comes in.

Imagine your body as a high-performance vehicle: Nutrition is the premium fuel that keeps the engine running smoothly, but even the best fuel won't matter if the car never goes in for maintenance. Sleep is that essential downtime when your body recharges, consolidates the benefits of good nutrition, and prepares you for the day ahead.

In the next chapter, we'll explore how sleep works hand in hand with nutrition to balance hormones, regulate hunger, and boost immunity. You'll learn why enough quality sleep isn't just about feeling rested it's a cornerstone of thriving health.

CHAPTER 6

E = Enough Sleep: The Rest You Deserve

The Power of Rest: Restorative Sleep: The Body's Repair System

Nothing heals the body more than uninterrupted sleep. We all need sleep to function! After focusing on oxygen, water, and nutrition, it's clear that the body is a finely tuned machine. But even the most well-maintained machine needs downtime to recharge and repair. Sleep is the missing piece in the puzzle of optimal health, completing the cycle of nourishment and restoration.

Sleep has a critical role in promoting health. The urgency of getting enough sleep cannot be overstated, as sleep is foundational for physical, mental, and emotional health. It's not merely a time of rest; it's when critical processes for repair, memory consolidation, and immune function occur.

Not getting enough sleep has been linked with a number of problems ranging from chronic disease to psychological problems. Research over the past decade has documented that sleep disturbance has a powerful influence on the risk of infectious disease, the occurrence and progression of several major medical illnesses including cardiovascular disease and cancer, anxiety and depression. Chronic sleep deprivation over time has even been linked to brain disorders such as schizophrenia and Alzheimer's.

Sleep's Role in Health

Our body rests, repairs and heals while we sleep, but we must have uninterrupted sleep for it to have the time it needs during sleep, the body undergoes processes that are crucial for survival and optimal function:

1. **Physical Healing**
   ○ Growth hormones are released during deep sleep, aiding in tissue repair, muscle development, and immune system strengthening.
2. **Memory and Learning**

- Sleep consolidates the day's experiences into long-term memory, sharpening focus and improving cognitive function.

3. **Hormone Regulation**
   - Sleep balances cortisol and insulin levels, which affect stress, metabolism, and inflammation.

4. **Immune Defense**
   - Antibodies and infection-fighting cells are produced during sleep, enhancing the body's ability to fight disease.

Consequences of Poor Sleep

The effects of chronic sleep deprivation are staggering, ranging from immediate fatigue to long-term health issues. Adults who sleep less than 7 hours per night are more likely to say they have had health problems, including heart attack, asthma, and depression, compared to those who get enough sleep (7 or more hours per night).

- **Physical Health**: Increased risk of diabetes, obesity, cardiovascular disease, and cancer.
- **Mental Health**: Anxiety, depression, and mood instability.
- **Cognitive Function**: Reduced memory, focus, and problem-solving ability.
- **Emotional Regulation**: Heightened stress and irritability.

In children, poor sleep can mimic ADHD symptoms, such as hyperactivity and difficulty focusing. Adults may experience low energy, cravings for sugar or caffeine, and slower reflexes.

When we do not get enough sleep and disrupt our circadian rhythm we do not give the body time to store our memories and rest our systems. This hinders our daily function the next day by roughly 35%. We wake up tired, have low energy, crave dopamine in the form of sugar or caffeine, and we do not think as clearly and our reflexes are slower. For our kids sleep deprivation creates hyperactivity and behavioral issues. We need efficient sleep to keep learning, functioning, and processing properly.

Sleep provides the body a chance to repair itself, boost the immune system, repair damaged tissues, grow muscles, retain memories and more.

Certain growth hormones are released during sleep only. Without adequate sleep, the body can't function properly and maintain itself.

Sleep actually provides "nutrition" to the brain. Sleeping too little causes the stress hormone cortisol to spike, signaling to your body to conserve more energy throughout the day. You're never getting into deep sleep, you stay in the light sleep. Even though you're in bed for 7 to 10 hours, you're not getting quality sleep. You stay in fight or flight, so you're not getting all the amazing hormones that are supposed to be released during deep sleep.

Cortisol makes you hyper during the day and increases anxiety and depression especially in young women. It increases inflammation. It prevents you from losing weight because we hold on to fat. Too much cortisol is bad for you.

If you're not breathing well, you can't reach deep sleep. If you're not reaching all of these stages, it's not healing. It's just breaking down every single day, affecting our bodies ability to function properly.

Bed wetting is the same survival mechanism. If your body is not able to breathe properly, and you know in a healthy way, your body kind of releases everything that's not important, some wet the bed, some will sweat.

Kids can be hyperactive due to lack of sleep and misdiagnosed with ADHD when they could have sleep disorder breathing (SDB) or sleep apnea. For it to be sleep apnea you have to stop breathing at least 10 seconds at a time in order for it to be considered an apnea. While a sleep study would show Apnea every single time that happens, it may not show arousals that are interrupting sleep in children. So a sleep study is not always recommended.

Arousals like a shift in brain activity or tossing and turning, kick you back to sleep stage one sleep, and you're not getting the benefits of sleep and oxygen.

So you're just starving yourself, your body, your cells and your organs.

In fact, some animals lose the ability to maintain their immune systems and die after experiencing weeks of sleep deprivation.

Extreme sleep deprivation messes with our immune response, causing an increase in inflammation across the body. When sleep becomes fragmented by easily preventable things, such as snoring and mouth breathing. It also causes a rise in blood pressure.

If you want to decrease sleep deprivation, addressing the root cause of sleep-disordered breathing that causes snoring, clenching and grinding is a great place to start.

As we've learned, the quality of our sleep is directly tied to the quality of our lives.

Mouth breathing at night causes snoring, which leads to poor oxygen exchange, fragmented sleep, and in severe cases, sleep apnea and other health conditions.

Proper airway health and breathing techniques can drastically improve our well-being. Putting an end to mouth breathing during the day requires some extra attention on our breathing, but what about at night when our subconscious mind takes over?

Since we can't actively pay attention to our breathing during sleep, the easiest way to ensure nasal breathing during rest is to tape your mouth shut before bed.

It's a proven solution that helps us get the adequate sleep we need to stay healthy and function properly.

During deep sleep, we don't expect to see any sort of airflow limitation. We shouldn't see any volume reductions during deep sleep. If we do, we know that there's an architecture problem, not enough room for the tongue and an airway or breathing issue.

When you put your child to sleep you might expect to hear a soft sigh or maybe a quiet buzz of a movie they fell asleep to, but one thing that parents do not want to hear is the sound of their child's teeth grinding together. Approximately three out of every ten children will grind or clench during their childhood years according to a Dr Kevin Boyd. While many children grow out of this habit with age, it can cause damage to the tooth enamel, chipped teeth, and can carry on into adulthood causing even greater problems.

Some children grind during the day when they are angry, stressed, or depressed, however, the majority of the time it occurs during sleep. Bruxism can leave your child waking up with earaches, headaches, and a sore jaw. Many parents do not even notice their child grinding their teeth because much of the grinding is done when the child is away in another room, out of the parents presence.

Staying attentive can give you great insight to learn if your child has Bruxism. Listen while they sleep, if you hear loud noises like rocks rubbing against each other, that is a good sign that your child is grinding their teeth. Other ways you can detect grinding is to take note when your child says he or she has a headache or sore jaw when they wake up.

Parents can work on reducing their child's stress before bedtime. By making them feel calm, relaxed and at ease, your child's grinding may also decrease. If the teeth grinding is in fact caused by stress, it is important to note that the grinding will not go away until the stress also goes away.

Understanding of the relationship between sleep, the neuroscience and autonomic pathways that connect sleep with the immune system is key to a happy healthy life.

The connection of the body and the mouth are a much under-discussed topic that need more awareness of what we can do early to prevent illnesses if we want to help our kids not suffer the same fate as their parents or grandparents.

You don't know what you don't know. I wish I knew this information sooner. I could have helped so many people. Knowing that I have learned about the connection, I made these changes to protect my daughter's future and the future of my grandchildren and great grandchildren from experiencing the same issues many people in my family have experienced. Some of which may be genetic but a lot are epigenetic.

Did you know that our motor and cognitive performance after staying awake for 24 hours is like having a blood alcohol level of 0.10%? At that level, we can expect to have significantly impaired motor coordination, loss of good judgment, slurred speech, impaired balance, vision, reaction time and hearing, and sensations of euphoria. Ever wonder why your kids are so revved up and slap happy when you know they're totally sleep-deprived and exhausted?

My daughter only cried when she was tired. So that is what made my mom instincts find another solution to what we were being told. Lack of sleep has so many health implications.

Have you ever considered kids diagnosed with ADHD may be sleep deprived? They have the same identical symptoms. If your child has an ADHD diagnosis consider an evaluation for sleep disorder breathing.

Strategies for improving sleep quality.

You know when your body and mind won't shut down as you go through your To-Do lists over and over in your head?

Or when you wake up in the middle of the night thinking about the same To-Do lists and just can't fall back asleep?

That's because cortisol, our stress hormone, is inappropriately surging at night and putting us in a "fight-or-flight" mode.

Here are the top 4 things you can do to get that good night's sleep!

Sleep routine

We all know that a good sleep routine is important. But what exactly is a "good" sleep routine? Here's a mnemonic to help you remember – **R.E.A.L**

- **R (Routine)** – establish regular sleep and wake up times. The sleep time between 9pm-5am is the most valuable, so adjust your sleep time according to your circadian rhythm. Go to bed only when sleepy and stay in bed only when asleep.

- **E (Environment)** – sleep in a dark quiet room with no pets; cool temperature, decrease EMF by turning off wifi, move cell phones 6 feet away from your bed,

  E is also for **Eating** – at least two hours before bed for a good night's sleep otherwise your body is busy digesting instead of resting and repairing.

- **A (Activity)** – do stimulating exercise early in the day and relaxing yoga exercises in the evening.

- **L (Light)** – dim lights and turn off or dim digital devices at least 2-3 hours before sleep.

Our "master clock" resets on a daily basis. It used to be by the sun rise and set.

Blue light tells our brain it's time to be awake, and melatonin secretion from our pineal gland tells us it's time to be asleep.

In nature, blue light occurs in the early morning to tell our brain to wake up and get ready for the day. Blue light is also emitted from most electronic screens (flat screen televisions, computers, laptops, smartphones and tablets) and fluorescent and LED lighting.

When we use any of these devices in the evening, our "master clock" is thrown off by as much as 3 hours, tricking our brains that it's daytime and making it nearly impossible to fall asleep at a reasonable hour.

We can do our part as parents, to limit screen time for our kids 2-3 hours before bedtime. Be sure to use blue light blocking glasses and screen dimming products to counteract this blue light effect on our sleep. Reading a book before bed is a good bedtime routine instead of a screen.

Hacks For Deep Sleep

1. Make sleep a priority

Sleep Deprivation is no joke! Sleep deprivation affects 50-70 million Americans, can lead to chronic illness, increase risks of diabetes, and heart attacks, and even reduce the production of cells which help to fight infection and cancer by 72%.

According to the World Health Organization (WHO), shift work disrupts the circadian rhythm and contributes to chronic illness due to lack of sleep. Our body repairs while we sleep. We were meant to go to sleep with the sunrise and sunset.

It's time to make sleep your priority!

2. Understand the science of sleep

Our body has 11 different systems all working together to keep us alive. Make it a habit to eat at least two hours before bed so the body is done digesting before you fall asleep.

How does our brain know when to start or end our sleep cycle?

How does our body adjust to different time zones or seasons?

Our circadian rhythm is the internal clock that guides our sleep-wake cycle. Our circadian rhythm is influenced by two main factors: external cues light and temperature and internal cues hormones and genes.

Our circadian rhythm can vary slightly from person to person, depending on their genetic makeup. This can affect their preferred sleeping and waking times.

Circadian rhythm can also be disrupted by factors such as jet lag, shift work, daylight saving time or artificial light exposure at night. These factors can cause our internal clock to be out of sync with the external clock, leading to problems such as insomnia, sleep apnea, daytime sleepiness, anxiety, mood disorders, irritability, and behavioral concerns in children.

Some people have a longer circadian rhythm (called "night owls"), while others have a shorter one (called "morning larks").

Have you ever heard the saying if you stay up with the owls you can't soar with the eagles? I don't know if that is true. But I do know lack of sleep affects cognitive ability the next day.

Action Steps:

To maintain a healthy circadian rhythm, follow these simple steps:

- Exposing yourself to bright light during the day, especially in the morning, 10 minutes of morning sun gives you more essential vitamin D.
- Getting around 6-8 hours of uninterrupted sleep per night for most adults, or 8 to 10 hours for most children.

- Make your bedroom dark, cool, quiet and comfortable, and use your bedroom for sleep only. No TV in the room preferably.
- Keeping a regular sleep schedule, going to bed and waking up at the same time (+- 30 min) every day.
- Avoid napping in the day if you have difficulty sleeping at night.

3. Exercise

Sleeping recharges your energy. Exercising makes you feel sleepy and regulates your sleep cycle. Some movement for at least 30 minutes daily can lead to much better sleep!

Your body temperature lowers 30-90 minutes after you exercise, which mimics the natural cooling process that happens before sleep, which can help facilitate sleep. Working out at least 1-2 hours before your bedtime can improve your sleep!

4. Before-sleep rituals

An hour before bed is the time you should not work. Instead do some creative work, spend time talking with your loved ones, or go out for a stroll.

Listen to soothing music (preferably instrumental): If you are tossing in your bed, it's most likely due to too many thoughts hovering around. This is because the logical aspect of your brain (left brain) is quite active and running. When you hear music (instrumental), it helps activate the right side of the brain and calm down too many thoughts, helping you to fall asleep.

Taking a shower before bed: Do you remember a routine of bathing before bed as a toddler? Water flowing over you not only refreshes the body but also relaxes the mind and lowers the core body temperature. Just make sure the water is not too cold or too hot an hour before sleeping.

5. Tackle your mind of these sleep killers

Have you wondered why you find it difficult to sleep? Most probably it's one of these:

- Anxiety or uncertainty, fear of the unknown.

- Overthinking about life, work or past conflicts.
- Stress about losing sleep itself.
- You ate too close to bedtime.
- You're too full or hungry.

There's something common in all of that. It's the inability to handle the racing mind! Thoughts and emotions keep flooding you over and do not allow your mind to sneak into sleep.

The brain releases chemicals (cortisol and adrenocorticotropic hormones) that trigger fight, flight or freeze responses when the mind is overwhelmed by stress, worry or overthinking. These chemicals make the heart beat faster and the blood pressure rises. They also keep the body in a state of high alert. In this state, the brain becomes more sensitive to any discomfort, which makes sleeping harder!

So how to halt this cycle? By learning to take control over the racing mind!

Find something that relaxes you before bed. Your subconscious likes to solve problems while you sleep. Give it a topic before bed so it is not finding one for you.

We live in a world dominated by screens, phones, tablets, computers, and TVs that have become an inescapable part of modern life. While they keep us connected and entertained, they also come with hidden costs for our sleep and overall health.

Blue Light and Sleep Disruption

Screens emit blue light, a high-energy wavelength that interferes with melatonin production, the hormone that regulates sleep. Exposure to blue light, especially in the evening, tricks your brain into thinking it's still daytime, delaying the natural onset of sleep. This disruption can lead to poor sleep quality, difficulty falling asleep, and long-term issues like fatigue and weakened immunity.

Poor Posture and Physical Health

Long hours spent hunched over screens lead to poor posture, often referred to as "tech neck." This strain affects the neck, shoulders, and spine, causing discomfort, reduced mobility, and even chronic pain. Over time, poor posture can also impair breathing, as slouched positions compress the chest and reduce lung capacity.

Cognitive and Emotional Impacts

Excessive screen time is also linked to increased stress, anxiety, and difficulty focusing. Constant alerts and notifications keep your brain in a heightened state of alertness, preventing you from fully relaxing, even when it's time to unwind.

Actionable Tips to Mitigate the Effects

1. **Limit Screen Time Before Bed**
   - Stop using screens at least 1–2 hours before bedtime to give your body time to wind down.
   - Use apps or device settings to enable night mode, which reduces blue light emissions.
2. **Invest in Blue Light Filters**
   - Consider wearing blue-light-blocking glasses if you work on screens for extended periods.
   - Use screen protectors or filters that reduce blue light exposure.
3. **Practice Good Posture**
   - Sit with your back straight, shoulders relaxed, and screen at eye level to avoid straining your neck.
   - Use ergonomic furniture, like chairs that support your back and desks at the correct height.
4. **Take Screen Breaks**
   - Follow the 20-20-20 rule: Every 20 minutes, look at something 20 feet away for 20 seconds.
   - Incorporate movement throughout your day by standing, stretching, or walking to reduce stiffness.
5. **Create a Sleep-Friendly Environment**
   - Keep your bedroom free of screens and distractions.

- Use blackout curtains and white noise machines to enhance sleep quality.
6. **Use Technology Wisely**
   - Set app limits or schedule downtime on your devices to reduce unnecessary usage.
   - Focus on mindful screen time by turning off non-essential notifications.

By being intentional about your screen habits, you can protect your sleep, posture, and overall well being. These small changes not only help you feel better physically but also allow you to stay more present and focused throughout your day.

Avoid these substances

Some substances can stimulate your nervous system and keep you awake or disrupt your sleep.

Caffeine can have a half-life of up to 6 hours, meaning that it can still affect your sleep even if you consume it in the afternoon.

Alcohol can make you feel sleepy at first, but it can also disrupt your sleep stages and cause waking up or nightmares.

Nicotine can also keep you alert and make it harder to fall asleep or stay asleep.

Don't eat heavy or spicy foods before bed. They can upset your stomach and ruin your sleep. Finish dinner at least 2-3 hours before bedtime. This gives your food time to digest and prevents acid reflux and other digestive issues.

Sleep pills can ruin your day with side effects like drowsiness, headache, nausea, and weakness. They can affect your driving, work, and social life and be addictive. Why risk it when you can sleep naturally? Try meditation, yoga, or breathing practices like pranayama to relax your body and mind and enjoy better, peaceful sleep.

If you do not sleep like a baby, you're not alone. Over 237 million people globally struggle to sleep well while 1 in 3 adults do not get enough sleep in the USA.

Controlling sleep environment, habits, and schedules can be helpful. But the most important skill required to sleep fast and deep is by taking complete control of your mind and emotions so that you can relax and get the sleep that you need!

Nutrients that help you sleep

Production of many of the neurotransmitters that regulate sleep depends on getting the right nutrients from our diet and supplements.

There are many supplements that can make sleep easier and more restful. Supplements that can assist with sleep are usually taken 1-2 hours before bedtime.

- Magnesium helps our minds to unwind and our muscles to relax. It also helps us to fall asleep faster by increasing melatonin levels and helps us to sleep longer!
- Chamomile tea is safe for all ages to help relax our bodies and minds and get ready for sleep.
- Melatonin is our sleep hormone. Melatonin supplementation can be helpful for better sleep.
- Drive by Aroga is here to help. Drive is the ONLY natural product that provides sustained energy and helps boost your mood. Once daily DRIVE provides nutrients that directly support apoptosis, autophagy, and mitochondria.
- Valerian root is the most studied herb for inducing sleep while promoting relaxation. However, it is not recommended during pregnancy and breastfeeding, and can taste quite strong. I use it in tea form before bed.

Reducing Stress is key

Stress reduction is key for a restorative night's sleep for you and your children.

The 20-minute Ultra Bath from UltraMind Solution by Dr. Mark Hyman is another great way to start the relaxation process at night. In the hottest water tolerable, combine 2 cups Epsom salts, 1 cup aluminum free baking soda, 10 drops lavender (halve this for a child). Epsom salts (which is magnesium sulfate) aid detoxification and also increase magnesium levels in our body.

Lavender relaxes our body and mind, decreases cortisol, and reduces inflammation. And hot water increases circulation and gets all those awesome Epsom salt and Lavender benefits flowing to all the parts of our body and brain.

Avoid stressful situations within 1 hour of bedtime that includes TV shows, video games, etc. and even bedtime conversations. Save stressful discussions for the daytime, and focus on positive and uplifting conversations before bedtime.

Read a book or sing goodnight songs with your children. Teach your children how to unwind through progressive relaxation, slow-paced belly breathing and nasal hygiene. End the night with gratitude by sharing 3 things that happened that day that you and your kids are grateful for. Send your children off to sleep with positive thoughts and feelings to fill their dreams and get ready for a beautiful new day.

So get into a good sleep routine, fill your body with the right nutrients, reduce stress – and get ready for a good night's sleep!

Early research and evidence indicates the possibility of repercussions that may impact growth and development and influence later diagnoses, such as attention deficit hyperactivity disorder (more commonly known as ADHD) due to lack of sleep in the pediatric population.

In theory if a child doesn't sleep well and the brain is not oxygenated well in early life, that individual may have morbidities diagnosed later in life, like anxiety, a learning or reading disability, or behavior problems.

Children don't normally report sleep issues. More often, the assessment is based on parents. But if the parents don't find a sleep issue (such as difficulty falling asleep or nighttime arousals) to be a concern or, more likely, they don't know about the child's sleep patterns because they are themselves sleeping, then it is likely to go unnoticed.

However, if parents are asked it is estimated that 80% will identify a sleep-related problem in their children. This doesn't mean that 80% of children have sleep disorders but it does indicate that we need to be more alert about sleepiness during the day and how it is affecting our kids. Approximately 25%

of all children experience some type of sleep problem at some point during childhood. Indicating the importance of focused screening.

There is significant need for additional education and support for primary care providers in the diagnosis and treatment of pediatric sleep disorders.

If you just look at growth and development, we know that sleep is a neurodevelopmental process, similar to walking and talking.

When a child is awake, stimulation comes from the environment. When asleep, it comes from dreaming. The brain is active during dream sleep, storing all of the memories from the day. If that sleep is interrupted, so is the process the body needs.

Sleep epidemic

Economic Impact.

Sleep deprivation costs the U.S. economy over $411 billion annually due to its impact on productivity and health care expenses.

These statistics underscore the critical roles that oxygen, water, nutrition, and sleep play in our health. They highlight not only the importance of each element on its own but also how they work together to support bodily functions and protect against disease.

Ensuring adequate intake and quality of these basic essentials can lead to better health outcomes, improved quality of life, and potentially a longer lifespan.

Sleep Studies and Testing: Your Guide to Proper Diagnosis

Why Sleep Studies Matter

During my years of practice, I've seen countless patients who were told their snoring was "normal" or that their child would "grow out of" their sleep issues. I was one of them. Another mother shared how her daughter had been diagnosed with ADHD, only to discover through proper sleep testing that the real issue was sleep-disordered breathing. This is why proper testing is crucial.

Types of Sleep Studies

1. Polysomnography (PSG) - In-Lab Sleep Study

This is considered the gold standard of sleep testing. However, there's something important you need to know - traditional sleep studies don't always tell the whole story, especially for children.

What's Measured:

- Brain waves (EEG)
- Eye movements
- Heart rate and rhythm
- Blood oxygen levels
- Breathing patterns
- Body movements
- Snoring intensity

Limitations to Consider:

- May not capture normal sleep patterns due to unfamiliar environment
- Might miss subtle breathing issues
- Often doesn't adequately assess children's sleep patterns
- Insurance may not cover without specific symptoms

2. Home Sleep Studies

These can be more comfortable and convenient, but have their own considerations.

Advantages:

- Natural sleep environment
- More affordable
- Easier for children
- Multiple night monitoring possible

Limitations:

- Less comprehensive data
- May miss certain sleep disorders

- Requires proper setup at home

3. Multiple Sleep Latency Test (MSLT)

This daytime test measures how quickly you fall asleep in a quiet environment during the day.

When It's Used:

- Diagnosing narcolepsy
- Evaluating excessive daytime sleepiness
- Following up on nighttime sleep studies

Warning Signs You Need a Sleep Study

Adults:

- Chronic snoring
- Witnessed breathing pauses
- Excessive daytime sleepiness
- Morning headaches
- Difficulty concentrating
- Mood changes
- High blood pressure
- Night sweats

Children:

- Bedwetting
- Night terrors
- Hyperactivity
- Dark circles under eyes
- Mouth breathing
- Behavioral issues
- Poor academic performance
- Morning headaches

Beyond Traditional Sleep Studies

Alternative Assessments:

- Airway evaluations
- Tongue and lip tie assessments
- Myofunctional evaluations
- Dental arch examinations

What to Expect During a Sleep Study

Before Your Sleep Study Action Steps to take for Success

Preparation Checklist:

1. Documentation to Gather:
   - Sleep diary (2 weeks minimum)
   - Symptom history
   - Medical history
   - Current medications
   - Family history
2. Physical Preparation:
   - Maintain normal sleep schedule
   - Avoid caffeine
   - List current supplements
   - Note any allergies
   - Document current symptoms
3. Insurance Preparation:
   - Verify coverage
   - Understand out-of-pocket costs
   - Get pre-authorization if needed
   - Know your deductible status

Preparation Steps

- Maintain normal daily routine
- Avoid caffeine after noon
- Bring comfortable sleepwear

- Pack toiletries
- List current medications
- Document recent sleep patterns

Required Items

- Insurance cards
- ID
- Sleep clothes
- Morning necessities
- Regular medications
- Completed questionnaires

During Your Sleep Study

Tips for Best Results:

1. Follow Your Normal Routine:
   - Stick to regular bedtime
   - Maintain usual hygiene practices
   - Bring comfortable sleepwear
   - Use your regular pillow
2. Documentation During Testing:
   - Note any unusual occurrences
   - Record time to fall asleep
   - Track nighttime awakenings
   - Monitor morning symptoms
3. Communication Guidelines:
   - Questions to ask technicians
   - When to alert staff
   - What to report

Monitoring Elements

1. Physical Measurements:
   - Brain waves
   - Heart rate
   - Breathing patterns

- Eye movements
- Muscle activity
- Oxygen levels
2. Environmental Factors:
   - Room temperature
   - Light levels
   - Sound monitoring
   - Position tracking

What It Feels Like

- Sensors are small and lightweight
- Wires are gathered to allow movement
- Room temperature is adjustable
- Staff available throughout night
- Normal bathroom breaks allowed

Common Concerns

Anxiety Management

- Staff is always available
- Communication system accessible
- Regular check-ins
- Adjustments possible
- Questions welcomed

Sleep Expectations

- First hour adjustment period
- Normal sleep not required
- Partial data still valuable
- Multiple positions allowed
- Natural wake-ups okay

After Your Sleep Study

- Schedule follow-up appointments
- Request complete test results

- Document any questions
- Note ongoing symptoms
- Understanding your numbers
- Identifying patterns
- Recognizing limitations
- Considering combinations of treatments
- Setting realistic expectations

Understanding Your Results

- Detailed report review
- Pattern identification
- Treatment options
- Recommendations
- Next steps

Interpreting Results

Common Terms and Measurements:
- Apnea-Hypopnea Index (AHI)
- Oxygen saturation levels
- Sleep efficiency
- Sleep stages

What's Being Missed

Many people suffer from undiagnosed sleep disorders, mistaking their symptoms for unrelated health issues. They also don't see getting up to pee as a disruption in sleep. It is in many cases diagnosed as a bladder issue not a breathing concern.

Sleep-Disordered Breathing (SDB) and Sleep Apnea

- **What's Missed:** Snoring, gasping, and frequent arousals disrupt sleep stages, leaving the body in a state of oxygen deprivation. Symptoms like fatigue, morning headaches, and **fragmented sleep** are often overlooked or dismissed as "normal."

- **What's Given:** C-pap machines, sleep appliances, exercises addressing airway issues, such as mouth breathing or nasal obstruction, can drastically improve sleep quality.

Mouth Breathing

- **What's Missed:** Mouth breathing reduces oxygen exchange, leading to snoring, dry mouth, dehydration and poor sleep quality.
- **What's Given:** Nasal hygiene, c-pap, myofunctional therapy, and in severe cases, tongue-tie release can help restore proper breathing patterns.

Teeth Grinding (Bruxism)

- **What's Missed:** Grinding and clenching during sleep can damage teeth, strain the jaw, and disrupt deep sleep stages.
- **What's Given:** Stress management, addressing airway issues, and correcting tongue posture, night guards or NTI's to protect teeth, and alleviate bruxism.

Sleep Quiz

Are you experiencing any of these sleep warning signs?

Instructions:

For each question, select the option that best describes your experience.

A=0 points   B=1 point   C=2 points   D=3 points

1. **Do you often breathe through your mouth, even when not exercising?**
   - A) Never
   - B) Sometimes
   - C) Frequently
   - D) Always
2. **Do you snore or have noisy breathing while sleeping?**
   - A) Never
   - B) Occasionally

- ○ C) Often
- ○ D) Every night

3. **Have you been diagnosed with sleep apnea or other sleep disorders?**
   - ○ A) No
   - ○ B) Not sure
   - ○ C) Suspected but not diagnosed
   - ○ D) Yes

4. **Do you have difficulty falling asleep or staying asleep?**
   - ○ A) Never
   - ○ B) Occasionally
   - ○ C) Frequently
   - ○ D) Always

5. **Do you experience bedwetting or getting up in the middle of the night to pee?**
   - ○ A) No
   - ○ B) Rarely
   - ○ C) Sometimes
   - ○ D) Often

6. **Are you often tired or sleepy during the day despite getting enough sleep at night?**
   - ○ A) Never
   - ○ B) Occasionally
   - ○ C) Frequently
   - ○ D) Always

7. **Do you have trouble focusing or paying attention, especially at work?**
   - ○ A) Never
   - ○ B) Sometimes
   - ○ C) Often
   - ○ D) Always

8. **Are you restless or tired during the day?**
   - ○ A) Never
   - ○ B) Occasionally

- ○ C) Frequently
- ○ D) Always

9. **Have you experienced delays in speech development or difficulty articulating words?**
   - ○ A) No
   - ○ B) Mild delays
   - ○ C) Noticeable delays
   - ○ D) Significant delays

10. **Do you have frequent ear infections or hearing problems?**
    - ○ A) Never
    - ○ B) Occasionally
    - ○ C) Often
    - ○ D) Always

11. **Do you have a narrow palate or crowded teeth?**
    - ○ A) No
    - ○ B) Slightly narrow
    - ○ C) Noticeably narrow
    - ○ D) Very narrow

12. **Do you have difficulty chewing, swallowing food or pills?**
    - ○ A) Never
    - ○ B) Occasionally
    - ○ C) Frequently
    - ○ D) Always

13. **Do you grind your teeth or clench your jaw at night?**
    - ○ A) Never
    - ○ B) Rarely
    - ○ C) Sometimes
    - ○ D) Often

Scoring:

- **0-7 Points:** You have a few, if any, myofunctional or breathing issues. Continue to monitor their habits and consult with a healthcare professional if you have any concerns.

- **8-19 Points:** You may have some signs of myofunctional or breathing issues. Consider seeking further evaluation to address these early and prevent potential complications.
- **20-29 Points:** You show multiple signs of myofunctional or breathing issues. It's important to consult with a myofunctional therapist or healthcare provider for a comprehensive evaluation and tailored intervention plan.
- **30+ Points:** You are likely experiencing significant myofunctional or breathing issues. Immediate consultation with a specialist is recommended to address these concerns and improve their health and wellbeing.

Remember: This quiz is not a diagnostic tool but can help you identify potential areas of concern. For a thorough evaluation and personalized advice, please consult with a myofunctional therapist or healthcare professional.

Sleep as an Urgent Priority

Sleep is not optional, it's a vital process that affects every aspect of health. Prioritizing quality sleep enables mental clarity, supports immune health, aids in physical recovery, and reduces the risk of chronic disease. Making sleep a non-negotiable part of your routine is an urgent and essential step toward a healthier, more balanced life.

Reaching Across Disciplines

We need more clinicians that can assess a sleep disorder. The identification of disordered sleep really rests on asking the right questions and being able to interpret the answers, and that really begins with all healthcare professionals.

We need a specialist to whom we can refer the patient if necessary. If you identify the problem but can do nothing about it, then the need for identification becomes questionable. Who do you get to help you? Finding practitioners who listen and don't tell you "your child will outgrow it", is difficult at the moment. We are not all on the same page.

Care also cannot be managed in isolation; it is a multidisciplinary approach. There are many dimensions and many disciplines involved that need to work together to identify those solutions that will impact children the most. These include (but are not limited to) child psychology, child psychiatry, pediatrician, pediatric otolaryngology, pediatric neurology, pediatric pulmonary medicine, pediatric dentist, oral surgery, chiropractor, speech pathologist, OT, PT, and myofunctional therapy.

Dr Kevin Boyd, DDS, MS, Dentistry for Children and Families, in Chicago, pediatric dentist offers training in sleep medicine risk assessment. Health professionals who frequently see children and can offer treatment options for some patients, particularly those diagnosed with sleep apnea and other airway ailments.

The sleep-specific education includes an assessment that incorporates parental interviews, patient responses, physical exam results, and risk factors, such as teeth grinding, snoring, chewing, swallowing, and specific physical features visible on x-ray images. Patients with suspected sleep apnea or other relevant conditions are sometimes then referred for sleep studies.

Here is another test we use to assess airway red flags

- Family history of sleep apnea
- Mouth-breathing
- Snoring, heavy, or noisy breathing while sleeping
- Restless sleep, waking up in a different position on the bed, or "bed clothes" are a mess
- Falling asleep at school or when riding in the care
- Chronic running or stuffy nose
- Dark circles under eyes or "allergic shiners"
- Night terrors
- Bedwetting
- Hard to wake up or tired in the morning
- Dry mouth at night and in the morning
- "Crooked" teeth and/or malocclusion
- Chronic ear infections
- Hyperactive behavior
- Sinusitis

If you or a loved one have any of these see an airway healthcare provider for next steps.

My Thoughts on Sleep

Sleep is the cornerstone of health, affecting everything from memory and mood to physical recovery and disease prevention. By understanding and addressing sleep issues, you can unlock better health, greater energy, and a higher quality of life. The power of quality sleep and its ability to restore and recharge the body is clear. Sleep is a profound act of self-respect. But here's the deeper truth: and the next pillar, respecting your body isn't just about how you sleep or what you eat, it's about recognizing that this is the one body you'll have for your entire journey through life.

Sleep is just one way we honor this incredible vessel, but respecting your body goes beyond any single habit. It's about embracing the idea that every choice you make, how you move, what you think, how you breathe reflects your commitment to your health.

Respecting your one body, not as a burden to maintain but as a gift to cherish, nurture, and protect.

Take the first step tonight: prioritize your sleep. It's not just an investment in yourself, it's a gift to your future.

CHAPTER 7

R = Respect: Self-Care, Stree, and the Vagus Nerve

The final pillar of health ties everything together: respecting yourself and your body. Respect begins with self-awareness, understanding what your body needs and continues with self-love, which drives your actions toward care and improvement.

To truly thrive, you must value yourself enough to prioritize your health. Respect is not just about taking care of your physical body; it's also about nurturing your emotional and mental well-being. Many of us live in survival mode, stuck in cycles of stress, burnout, and self-neglect, making decisions based on emotions rather than awareness.

Thoughts are the foundational role of self-love in building self-respect, the importance of regulating your nervous system, and how the vagus nerve serves as the bridge between emotional and physical health.

Yoga, stretching, and mindful movement are powerful practices that support both physical and mental health. Gently moving and stretching the body helps improve flexibility, posture, and joint mobility while reducing tension and stiffness in muscles. Beyond the physical benefits, movement promotes relaxation and stress relief by calming the nervous system and encouraging deep, intentional breathing. Regular practice can enhance circulation, boost energy levels, and support a healthy mind-body connection, making it a perfect way to reset and recharge. By connecting the mind, mouth and body through respect, you create the conditions for optimal wellness.

The Power of Self-Love and Respect

What is Self-Love?

Self-love is the act of accepting and valuing yourself unconditionally. It's about recognizing your worth, treating yourself with kindness, and understanding that you deserve care and respect just as much as anyone else. The thoughts we tell ourselves or beliefs. Words matter whether we say them outloud or not.

Many of us prioritize the needs of others, neglecting our own well-being in the process. But here's the truth: you cannot pour from an empty cup. To give love and support to others, you must first give it to yourself.

Learning to Respect Myself

For years, I believed I could handle anything. I was the problem-solver, the caretaker, the person everyone else leaned on. But I didn't realize how much of myself I was giving away and how little I was keeping for myself.

During my divorce, I was juggling everything: my job, my child, sleep and the emotional weight of trying to keep it all together. I told myself I didn't have time to rest or ask for help. I pushed through the stress, ignoring the warning signs my body was giving me.

It wasn't until my cancer diagnosis that I finally had to stop and face the truth. My body wasn't just breaking down overnight; it had been sending me signals for years. The constant stress, the sleepless nights, and the inability to say "no" had taken their toll.

One of the first signs I ignored was my bleeding gums. As a dental professional, I knew what that could mean, but I dismissed it. I was too busy to address it and convinced myself it wasn't important. But looking back, I realize it was my body's way of telling me something was wrong something bigger than I could see.

That diagnosis forced me to reassess everything. My body wasn't failing me; I had failed to respect it. The stress I carried, the neglect I tolerated, and the refusal to prioritize my own needs had created the perfect storm.

What I Learned

Looking back, I now understand how deeply stress and self-sabotaging thoughts and neglect for myself were tied to my health. The constant state of fight-or-flight weakened my immune system, and the lack of self-care and sleep left me vulnerable.

Cancer was my wake-up call, but it shouldn't take a life-altering diagnosis for us to realize the importance of self-respect.

I began to make small changes at first. I started saying no when I needed to. I prioritized rest and stopped apologizing for taking time for myself. I began treating my body like an ally instead of an afterthought.

Respecting yourself isn't selfish, it's survival. And it's the foundation for everything else: your health, your relationships, and your ability to thrive.

Signs You May Struggle with Self-Love

1. **Negative Self-Talk**: Criticizing yourself more harshly than you would anyone else.
2. **Overworking**: Believing your value comes from productivity rather than who you are and how you feel.
3. **Difficulty Setting Boundaries**: Saying yes to others at the expense of your own needs.
4. **Ignoring Your Body's Signals**: Pushing through fatigue, pain, or stress without addressing it.

The Vagus Nerve: The Mind-Body Connection

While self-love forms the foundation of self-respect, the vagus nerve provides the mechanism for regulating your emotional and physical states.

What is the Vagus Nerve?

The vagus nerve is the 10th cranial nerve and the longest nerve in the body. It connects your brain to your heart, lungs, gut, and other vital organs. It is a key player in the parasympathetic nervous system, responsible for the "rest and digest" state that allows your body to recover and heal.

Functions of the Vagus Nerve:

- **Calms Stress Responses**: Activates relaxation after stress or danger.
- **Improves Digestion**: Stimulates the gut to produce enzymes and move food through efficiently.
- **Supports Heart Health**: Helps regulate heart rate and blood pressure.

- **Balances Emotions**: Enables communication between the brain and gut, influencing mood and mental health.

The Problem: Living in Fight-or-Flight Mode

Many people live in a constant state of stress, or sympathetic dominance, where the fight-or-flight response takes over. This can lead to:

- Anxiety and irritability.
- Digestive problems.
- Chronic fatigue.
- Difficulty concentrating.

When the vagus nerve is not functioning well, you may feel stuck in this state, unable to fully relax or recover. Improving vagal tone can restore balance and promote resilience.

Self-Assessment: Is Your Nervous System Out of Balance?

Rate each symptom on a scale of 0–4:

- 0 = Never
- 1 = Rarely
- 2 = Sometimes
- 3 = Often
- 4 = Constantly

Physical Symptoms

- Sleep disruption: _____
- Digestive issues: _____
- Racing heart: _____
- Muscle tension: _____
- Fatigue: _____

Emotional Symptoms

- Anxiety or worry: _____
- Difficulty focusing: _____
- Mood swings: _____
- Feeling overwhelmed: _____

Behavioral Patterns

- Avoiding situations: _____
- Overreacting to stress: _____
- Procrastination: _____
- People-pleasing: _____

What Your Score Means:

- **Mild (0–10)**: Your nervous system is relatively balanced. Maintain good habits to stay resilient.
- **Moderate (11–25)**: Your nervous system is under stress. Implement calming practices to restore balance.
- **Severe (26+)**: Your nervous system needs immediate attention. Seek professional support to address underlying issues.

Strengthening the Vagus Nerve

Improving vagal tone can help your body shift out of fight-or-flight mode and into a state of relaxation.

Techniques to Improve Vagal Tone

1. **Deep Breathing**
   - Inhale deeply through your nose for 4 seconds, hold for 4 seconds, and exhale slowly for 8 seconds.
2. **Cold Exposure**
   - Splash cold water on your face or end your shower with 30 seconds of cold water.
3. **Humming or Chanting**
   - The vibrations stimulate the vagus nerve and activate relaxation.
4. **Mindful Meditation**
   - Spend 5–10 minutes focusing on your breath or repeating a calming mantra.

Respect as the Key to Wellness

Respecting yourself isn't just about making healthier choices, it's about recognizing how every part of your body works together to support overall health. This includes areas we often overlook, like oral health. Your mouth is more than a tool for eating and speaking; it's a gateway to your entire body's health. By understanding and caring for your oral health, you unlock another essential piece of the puzzle for creating a balanced, resilient, and vibrant life. The connection between your mouth and your body is profound, and it's a connection that truly deserves your attention.

CHAPTER 8

Oral Health: The Mouth Body Connection

Your Mouth, Your Health

Oral health is not just about teeth it's about understanding how your mouth, tongue, and oral habits impact your overall health. From your breathing to your sleep, to your posture and systemic health, the mouth is the gateway to your entire body. Addressing oral health holistically can transform not only your physical well-being but also your emotional health and quality of life.

The Mouth: Gateway to the Body

The mouth processes food, enables speech, and serves as the entry point for nutrients and potentially harmful pathogens. When bacteria, toxins, or other pathogens slip past the body's defenses, they can enter the bloodstream and wreak havoc.

But oral health isn't just about fluoride and avoiding cavities. It involves maintaining balance across multiple components:

- Teeth and gums
- Tongue and saliva
- Roof of the mouth and throat
- Mouth pH and breathing habits

Your oral health is directly connected to systemic issues like inflammation, breathing disorders, digestion, and even mental health.

The mouth is our gateway to the rest of the body, a pathway for everything that passes through it. Sometimes pathogens and toxins slip through the body's many defense mechanisms and hang around, when you brush they can enter the bloodstream. Good oral hygiene and proper breathing are an important component to maintaining a healthy balance in the mouth. But there is so much more.

A healthy mouth is more than just preventing cavities, gingivitis and gum disease, the health of your mouth is directly related to the overall health of your body. For ultimate health your oral health habits should include everything in your mouth from teeth, gums, tongue, saliva, tissues, roof of your mouth, throat and pH, to what you put in your mouth.

Most dental professionals are taught to teach our patients to brush, floss and avoid sugar, use a fluoridated toothpaste and visit the dentist twice a year. Unfortunately many patients have followed these practices and are discouraged when they are doing all of this and are still getting cavities and dental disease.

Most of us grow up seeing a medical doctor to take care of our bodies and a dentist to take care of our mouth.

When I first became a dental hygienist, I was taught to review the patient's medical history to ensure that there was no medical condition, allergies or medication that would affect the patient's dental care and/or treatment. I looked to see if there was anything in their mouth that I needed to know that would affect treatment that day. I charted the information, cleaned their teeth and informed the dentist of my findings.

There is minimal communication between the medical doctor and the dentist in providing dental care to a patient. This has always been something that I never understood.

I started seeing patterns. This is when I started to put it all together. Also, I had so many things happening in my own life, I was seeing the mind-mouth-body connection.

What I was finding in talking to parents and caregivers was we are not very knowledgeable in caring for our teeth. Over the past thirty years working in different dental settings I found that what patients are taught as a consumer depends on the knowledge, beliefs and education of the provider they are seeing. I was one of those provided that had no clue the extent our mouth played in our overall health.

Many people believe sensitive teeth, bleeding gums, cavities and tooth loss are inevitable. It is in their genes or that soft teeth run in their family. That cannot be further from the truth. No disease is inevitable, it is our mindset, beliefs, circumstances, and habits that affect our health.

So what now? Who do you seek help from?

You need to know your wants, needs and your beliefs so you can make informed decisions that are right for you, the health of your mouth and the long term health of your body. Pick a provider that has a similar mindset and ask a lot of questions.

Damaged teeth and gums can be reversed under certain conditions, if caught soon enough. We create the conditions in our body. We can uncreate them if we have illnesses, or we can prevent them from happening in the first place.

For teeth, natural tooth enamel can repair itself and heal a soft spot before it breaks through the surface of the tooth to the middle layer. So when does a tooth require a filling? That is a subject of great debate that depends on the dentist you see, their education and beliefs. One dentist may fill a dark spot, another will put a watch on it till the next visit, while another may suggest you use a method to rebuild and strengthen the tooth with fluoride, xylitol or other products.

Not all dentists believe in natural repairs at home. Let's face it, not all patients will follow an at home routine and the problems progress.

So what is the correct answer? Fortunately new technology helps patients have more choices. It is not a simple answer and has many factors at play: your beliefs, the dentist's beliefs, your medical history, your oral hygiene, your diet, the pH of your mouth, your budget and the time you have to invest in your mouth.

If you choose the repair at home method, it is on you, not the dental professional. This is why these methods are not the mainstream; it is out of the control of the treating dentist. We are all responsible for the choices we make. The problem is that we have limited information when we make many of these choices.

When I was little we were taught you should brush three times a day, floss and visit a dentist twice a year. When I went to hygiene school we were taught to brush twice a day, floss, use a fluoride toothpaste, mouth rinse and visit your dentist. You see a dentist for your mouth and teeth and a doctor for your body health. Now I know just how connected they are. Your mouth gives you warning signs and you should be looking at your tongue, how it functions, how you breathe, your habits and mindset.

Times are changing with more research linking the health of your mouth to different diseases in the body. It is all connected. We need to start looking at it and treating it that way.

When I graduated dental hygiene school I won a fellowship to study at Micheal Reese hospital in Chicago. I was so excited to learn as much as I could about how your mouth is connected and what we were telling patients from a medical viewpoint. One day I was working in the Cancer unit, the doctor was talking to a patient about treatment. After he finished writing his notes in the chart, I chimed in with what to expect in her mouth while going through chemo, how saliva reduces and she could be more susceptible to cavities and gingivitis. Recommended what she could do to lessen the chances of that happening. I quickly learned I was there to observe and not offer advice. It was very disheartening to me when the patient left and the doctor told me we were not there to care about her mouth.

He was saving her life. I said a simple conversation can prevent her from having to have major dental work after you save her life. Why not take the time and save her from having to go through something that could be prevented? I quickly learned my place. I also let that shut me down instead of speaking up. I just graduated, what did I know? It took years before we started telling them how to keep their teeth healthy when going through chemo and radiation.

I have always believed your mouth was connected to the rest of your body, but after that experience I questioned myself instead of speaking up and talking about it, I needed more than just a feeling I needed proof, for the longest time I felt like I was fighting an uphill battle. It has taken years, now we have the proof and the medical community agrees there is a connection.

I am happy that we now explain to patients what to expect in their mouths during radiation and chemo treatments. In some cases we even see patients before they have treatment so they know where they stand, what they can expect and how to keep their mouth healthy during treatment.

If you have poor oral health or chronic inflammation in your mouth it can increase your risk of heart disease, heart attack, stroke, diabetes, Alzheimer's, dementia, preterm delivery or low birth weight, and certain forms of cancer.

Inflammation in your mouth could be a warning sign to you if you have not been diagnosed with one of these things. We have sent patients to their physician to get tested after not being able to get their bleeding gums under control and they have been diagnosed with things like diabetes, leukemia, thyroid problems, even cancer.

My uncle lost teeth and struggled with gum disease. When we sent him to get blood work they said everything was normal. No matter what treatment we tried we could not get his inflamed bleeding gums under control. Five years later he was diagnosed with diabetes. Once he got his sugar under control his gums got better. I have seen it time and time again with other patients.

Three years later his gums started bleeding again, he was told everything was ok. It really does depend on your healthcare provider, how much you listen to the warning signs, what treatment you receive. By the time he was diagnosed with his cancer he was in stage four. This is why I am such an advocate about how your mouth is connected to your overall health.

I truly believe if I was more vocal about what I was seeing and feeling we could have gotten him help sooner. It is hard to know what the right thing to do is, especially when the doctor's back then did not believe what you were saying.

A Hard Lesson Revisited

Fast forward 30 years. I had since been diagnosed with cancer, and later, my father faced the same battle. Once again, during my treatment, no one mentioned oral health. Even though I knew the connection, having discovered my own cancer partly because of bleeding gums there was no guidance about how my treatment might affect my mouth or what I could do to mitigate these effects.

Why was I surprised? The healthcare system continues to treat oral health as a separate issue. While some progress has been made in educating people about the mouth-body connection, it's still not enough.

The impact of poor oral health on overall health is not completely understood. Saliva, diet, pH, blood chemistry all need to be monitored and patients should be their own health care advocates. Knowledge and education is the best way to prevent disease from happening.

If you begin a preventive program, maintain good oral habits, visit the dentist regularly and consult your physician for yearly blood work, especially if things are out of balance, you can avoid most if not all dental problems in the future.

The fundamental elements of health, oxygen, water, nutrition, and sleep are often discussed separately but are interconnected in maintaining and improving overall health and well-being.

While these elements are crucial the function of your tongue plays a huge role in meeting the above needs.

The Tongue: A Vital Mighty Yet Overlooked Muscle

The tongue is one of the most underrated yet powerful parts of our body. Often overlooked, this small organ plays a significant role in our health and well-being.

Understanding its anatomy, functions, and potential issues early in life can be a game-changer for your family.

Is Your Tongue the Culprit Behind Your Health Problems?

When it comes to health, we often scrutinize our diet, exercise, and lifestyle choices, but how often do we consider the role of our tongue? Yes, you heard it right — your tongue!

This often-overlooked organ could be silently influencing your overall health in ways you might not have imagined.

Understanding the Tongue's Impact

The tongue plays a crucial role in our oral ecosystem. It's not just essential for taste and speech; it also has significant implications for our dental and overall health.

- **Oral Health:** The texture and cleanliness of your tongue can affect your mouth's health. A coated tongue, for instance, can harbor bacteria and contribute to bad breath and tooth decay.
- **Digestive Health:** Digestion starts in the mouth, and the tongue is a key player. A healthy tongue aids in the proper mastication and breakdown of food, which is vital for optimal digestion.
- **Respiratory Issues:** A mispositioned tongue can lead to mouth breathing, which has been associated with snoring and sleep apnea, conditions that significantly impact sleep quality and overall health.

Signs Your Tongue Might Be Causing Trouble

- White Coating: This could indicate an overgrowth of bacteria or yeast.
- Persistent Bad Breath: Bacteria on the tongue can produce foul-smelling compounds.
- Change in Texture or Color: These changes can be signs of nutritional deficiencies or other health issues.
- Difficulty Swallowing or Speaking: These could be symptoms of an underlying neuromuscular issue.
- Open bite or tongue thrust swallow: Meaning there is a space between your teeth when you bite and your tongue may slide through it when you swallow.

The Tongue-Body Connection

The state of your tongue can be a window to your general health. Traditional practices like Ayurveda and Chinese medicine have long used tongue diagnosis as a method to detect imbalances in the body. While this method is not used in modern medical diagnosis, it does highlight the tongue's relevance in overall health monitoring.

If you notice you are having difficulty sleeping, waking up, dry mouth, chapped lips, persistent changes in the appearance or function of your tongue, it's important to consult a healthcare professional. They can help determine if these changes are indicative of a deeper health issue.

Trouble breathing, thinking, tired all the time? Breathing through your mouth, not your nose?

How much do you think about your tongue?

What do you really know about the tongue?

Do you know just how important your tongue is to the health of your body?

Your mouth is a window into the body and your tongue is the managing director!

Where is your tongue? Who is really in charge? You or your tongue?

Where is it resting in your mouth up, down or somewhere in the middle? Are you muscle bracing? Is your tongue relaxed or are you pushing it up or to the sides of your teeth?

When you stick your tongue out do you have indentations on the sides known as scalloping?

Discover how your tongue interacts with your overall health.

Discuss what you can do to help yours and your families health. This is genetic and usually one or more family members are struggling and have no idea their tongue position and posture is the issue.

Habits are something you can change. What is your habit with your tongue? Take some time and evaluate it. When you open wide can you touch the roof of your mouth without closing? If not your tongue may not be functioning properly.

This is one reason why you might find it hard to wake up or wake up feeling tired, when you wake up you find yourself falling back asleep. Your brain values oxygen and its long-term benefits are something you need nasal breathing for, but it values immediate gratification when it comes to the present moment. Mouth breathing when you are sleeping may be a habit. Time to make a change in your life.

Fascinating Facts About the Tongue

The tongue plays a critical role in speech, swallowing, breathing, and maintaining oral posture. Its resting position and function can affect everything from your jaw alignment to your ability to sleep and breathe properly.

Fascinating Facts About the Tongue

- The average tongue is about 3 inches long.
- It's the only muscle in the body that is attached at only one end.
- The tongue has 8 muscles that intertwine with each other, allowing for its incredible flexibility and strength.
- An adult has between 2,000 to 4,000 taste buds, and they regenerate approximately every two weeks.
- We swallow 800- 2000 times a day with one to six pounds of pressure on the surrounding structures.
- Form follows function so how our tongue functions determines how our face grows.

Anatomy of the Tongue

The tongue is a muscular organ and consists of two main parts:

1. **Body:** The visible part, which you can move around.
2. **Root:** The part that attaches to the floor of the mouth.

Here are the details of the tongue's anatomy and the eight muscles that allow it to move in various directions up, down, side to side, and even in a circular motion, that make it such a versatile and powerful organ.

These movements are crucial for function, speaking, eating, swallowing, breathing, and sleeping. The surface of the tongue is covered with tiny bumps called papillae, which house taste buds. These taste buds are responsible for detecting different flavors—sweet, salty, sour, and bitter.

These muscles are categorized into two groups: intrinsic and extrinsic. Each muscle plays a specific role in the tongue's movement and function, allowing us to speak, eat, and swallow effectively.

Intrinsic Muscles

The intrinsic muscles are located entirely within the tongue. They are responsible for altering the shape of the tongue, such as curling, flattening, and elongating. There are four intrinsic muscles:

1. **Superior Longitudinal Muscle:**
   - ○ **Location:** Runs along the top of the tongue from front to back.
   - ○ **Function:** Elevates the tongue tip, assists in retraction, and helps shape the tongue.
2. **Inferior Longitudinal Muscle:**
   - ○ **Location:** Runs along the bottom of the tongue from front to back.
   - ○ **Function:** Lowers the tongue tip and assists in retraction.
3. **Transverse Muscle:**
   - ○ **Location:** Runs horizontally across the tongue.
   - ○ **Function:** Narrows and elongates the tongue, which is crucial for swallowing and speech articulation.
4. **Vertical Muscle:**
   - ○ **Location:** Runs vertically from the top to the bottom surface of the tongue.
   - ○ **Function:** Flattens and broadens the tongue, aiding in the creation of a wide surface area.

Extrinsic Muscles

The extrinsic muscles originate outside the tongue and attach to it. They are responsible for the tongue's overall movement within the mouth. There are four extrinsic muscles:

1. **Genioglossus:**
   - ○ **Location:** Originates from the mandible (lower jawbone) and inserts into the tongue.
   - ○ **Function:** Protrudes the tongue and helps depress the center of the tongue. It's the primary muscle used for sticking out the tongue.
2. **Hyoglossus:**
   - ○ **Location:** Originates from the hyoid bone and inserts into the sides of the tongue.
   - ○ **Function:** Depresses and retracts the tongue, contributing to the downward movement.

3. **Styloglossus:**
   - ○ **Location:** Originates from the styloid process of the temporal bone and inserts into the sides of the tongue.
   - ○ **Function:** Retracts and elevates the tongue, playing a role in swallowing.
4. **Palatoglossus:**
   - ○ **Location:** Originates from the soft palate and inserts into the sides of the tongue.
   - ○ **Function:** Elevates the back of the tongue and depresses the soft palate, important for the initiation of swallowing.

These muscles and their functions highlight just how well-coordinated our tongue's movements are. The muscles work together seamlessly, allowing us to perform essential tasks.

Understanding the tongue's anatomy, functions, and potential issues allows us to appreciate its importance and take better care of it. When they do not function properly it can have an effect on speaking clearly, chewing efficiently, swallowing safely, our ability to taste, digest food properly, behavior, sleep, snoring and more.

A healthy properly functioning tongue plays a crucial role in our overall well-being.

Functions of the Tongue

The tongue is a multi-functional organ, crucial for various tasks:

1. **Taste:** Taste buds on the tongue help us enjoy and notice different flavors.

2. **Speech:** The tongue's movements are essential for expressing sounds and words.
3. **Chewing and Swallowing:** Helps with stimulating saliva, forming a bolus, preparing and digesting food, pushing it towards the throat for swallowing.
4. **Cleaning:** The tongue naturally cleanses the mouth by removing food particles and bacteria from the teeth and folds of the mouth.

Common Tongue Issues and Restrictions

Tongue-Tie (Ankyloglossia): One of the most common issues is tongue-tie, a condition where the tissue connecting the tongue to the floor of the mouth (the frenulum) is too short or tight. This can restrict the tongue's movement, affecting function, breastfeeding in infants, breathing, sleep, speech development in children, and even oral hygiene in adults.

Geographic Tongue: This is a harmless condition where patches on the tongue are red or white, giving it a map-like appearance. While it's generally painless, some parts of the tongue lose the papillae; and can sometimes cause discomfort or sensitivity to certain foods.

Oral Thrush: Is a fungal infection caused by Candida yeast, leading to white patches on the tongue and inner cheeks. It's more common in infants, the elderly, or in individuals with weakened immune systems.

Tongue Cancer: May have a white or red appearance, persistent sores, lumps, or pain. Early detection is key to successful treatment.

Caring for Your Tongue

Maintaining a healthy tongue is vital for overall oral health. Here are some tips:

1. **Good Oral Hygiene:** Brush your tongue gently with a toothbrush or a tongue scraper to remove bacteria and debris.
2. **Stay Hydrated:** Drink plenty of water to keep your mouth moist and help prevent bacterial overgrowth.
3. **Healthy Diet:** Avoid excessive sugar and acidic foods that can create inflammation.

4. **How does it function:** The resting position and function of the tongue are key to overall health and not something that is common to evaluate. This should be one of the first things we look at in our children. Tongue ties and tethered tissues are hereditary. Not all need to be treated. There is alot to consider. Which will be addressed in another chapter.

Remember to give your tongue the attention it deserves, appreciating your tongue and all it does for you! Your mouth and your entire body are all connected and function systematically.

When we know better we can do better. Or do we?

Common knowledge does not always mean common practice.

Knowing does not always = doing. This is a guideline to understand how everything is connected and how simple shifts in habits can make a huge difference.

More about the role of the tongue and its function later.

Is Your Tongue in the Proper Resting Position?

Back to the tongue function. The tongue's proper positioning is crucial. When it doesn't rest or function correctly, it can disrupt the airway, impacting both physical and mental health. Surprisingly, approximately 50% of Americans have improper tongue posture, a condition often overlooked despite its profound effects on the body.

Where Should Your Tongue Rest?

Take a moment to notice: where is your tongue right now?

- Is it lying at the bottom of your mouth?
- Floating somewhere between your teeth?
- Or suctioned against the roof of your mouth?

If your answer is suctioned to the roof of your mouth, congratulations! That's where it should be 24/7—unless you're eating or talking.

Proper Tongue Positioning

Known as oral rest posture, the correct resting position for your tongue is against the roof of your mouth. It should not press against the back of your front teeth, and your teeth should remain slightly apart. Your lips should close naturally over your teeth without straining.

Improper tongue positioning, on the other hand, can lead to a host of issues, including:

- Jaw and neck pain
- Breathing difficulties
- Sleep disturbances
- Misaligned teeth
- Poor posture

Signs of Improper Tongue Positioning

If you're unsure whether your tongue is in the right place, here are some common signs of poor tongue posture:

- Chronic mouth breathing
- Teeth grinding or jaw clenching
- Neck, shoulder, or jaw pain
- Snoring or sleep apnea
- Frequent fatigue or waking up unrefreshed
- Misaligned teeth
- Habitual poor posture
- Dark circles under the eyes

Correcting Tongue Positioning

Awareness is the first step. Throughout your day, check in with your tongue and ask:

- Is it pressing against the back of your teeth or lying passively in your mouth?
- Are your lips frequently open? This could indicate mouth breathing, often a sign of poor tongue posture.

If improper tongue positioning persists, you may need professional help. Myofunctional therapy, orthodontic evaluation, or other treatments can correct the issue and prevent long-term complications.

Picky Eating: More Than a Phase

For many parents, picky eating can feel like a frustrating phase. But what if it's not just about preferences or habits? What if the root cause lies in your child's tongue and how it functions?

Children with oral restrictions, such as tongue-tie or improper tongue posture, often struggle with certain textures and foods. Foods that are hard to chew, like meats or raw vegetables, can feel impossible to manage when the tongue isn't moving effectively. These struggles can quickly lead to food aversions and reinforce a limited diet.

The Role of the Tongue in Eating

The tongue is essential for breaking food into manageable pieces and coordinating the swallow. When it doesn't function properly, your child may:

- Prefer soft, processed foods over fibrous or crunchy options.
- Gag or choke on foods with specific textures.
- Avoid trying new foods, leading to nutritional gaps.

Additionally, sensory sensitivities often accompany tongue dysfunction. This means children may find certain textures overwhelming or even distressing, compounding their picky eating habits.

When to Seek Help

If picky eating persists or is accompanied by difficulty chewing, gagging, or swallowing, it's worth consulting a professional. Myofunctional therapy, combined with an evaluation for tongue-tie or oral-motor dysfunction, can provide targeted solutions. These therapies can:

- Improve tongue mobility, making eating less of a challenge.
- Desensitize oral sensitivities, allowing children to explore new foods.
- Support the development of a balanced, nutrient-rich diet.

How Parents Can Help

While therapy is essential for addressing the root cause, parents can support their children with simple strategies at home:

- Gradually introduce new textures by blending favorite foods with small amounts of new ones.
- Encourage chewing exercises to strengthen oral muscles.
- Create a low-pressure mealtime environment to reduce stress.

What Is a Tongue Thrust Swallow?

A tongue thrust swallow, also known as an infantile or reverse swallow, is a condition where the tongue pushes forward against the front teeth during swallowing instead of pressing against the roof of the mouth.

While common in infants, most children outgrow this pattern by the age of 6 or 7. However, if it persists into adulthood, it can lead to:

- Dental misalignment (open bites or overbites)
- Speech difficulties
- Sleep disturbances
- Behavioral issues

Contributing Factors

Several factors can contribute to tongue thrust swallow, including:

- Prolonged oral habits, like pacifier use or thumb sucking
- Tethered oral tissues, such as tongue-tie, which restricts the tongue's movement
- Structural issues, like a vaulted palate, that limit tongue function

Treatment Options

1. Tongue Exercises: Strengthen the tongue and retrain its movement with guided exercises.
2. Myofunctional Therapy: Focuses on retraining the muscles of the face, tongue, and mouth.

3. Orthodontic Treatment: Corrects dental issues caused by tongue thrust, such as misaligned teeth.
4. Behavior Modification: Breaking habits like nail-biting or excessive gum-chewing can support recovery.

For complex cases, a team approach involving dentists, speech-language pathologists, orthodontists, chiropractor, and more may be necessary.

The Role of Tongue-Ties

A tongue-tie, or ankyloglossia, occurs when the (Facia) tissue connecting the tongue to the floor of the mouth is too tight, limiting its range of motion. This condition can cause:

- Difficulty breastfeeding in infants
- Speech delays in children
- Oral hygiene challenges and sleep issues in adults

Posterior tongue-tie, a subtler form of the condition, often goes undiagnosed but can still lead to significant functional problems.

Complications of Untreated Tongue Issues

If left untreated, tongue-related issues can result in:

- Misaligned teeth: Caused by constant pressure from the tongue.
- Sleep apnea: Due to airway obstruction.
- Chronic pain: In the neck, jaw, and shoulders.
- Behavioral challenges: Especially in children.

The Tongue-to-Toe Connection

Have you ever heard the children's song *"Dem Bones"*? It describes how everything in the body is interconnected:

The toe bone's connected to the foot bone...

What you might not know is that your tongue is connected to your toes!

This connection exists through a network of connective tissue called fascia, a thin, web-like tissue that wraps around muscles, nerves, and blood vessels throughout the body. When the tongue is out of place, it can disrupt the balance of this entire system, causing effects that ripple all the way down to your toes.

The Fascia Web: Myofascial Meridians and Compensation Patterns

Imagine your body is wrapped in a continuous, elastic web of connective tissue called fascia, a structure that supports and integrates every muscle, organ, and bone. This web isn't just a passive scaffold; it's alive, responsive, and deeply interconnected, forming pathways called myofascial meridians that link distant parts of the body.

The Myofascial Meridians: A Highway of Connection

Myofascial meridians, also known as anatomy trains, are lines of connective tissue (fascia) that run throughout the body, linking muscles and bones into functional units. They help in understanding how movement and tension are distributed across the body.

These meridians, or lines of tension, act like highways through which strain, movement, and compensation travel. For instance:

- The **deep front line** runs from the tongue and jaw down through the neck, chest, diaphragm, spine, and into the pelvis and legs, even extending to the toes.
- A dysfunction in one area, such as a restricted tongue or tight jaw, can create imbalances along the entire chain, manifesting as poor posture, chronic pain, or limited mobility elsewhere in the body.

When Fascia is Tight: Compensation in Action

Tight or restricted fascia doesn't just create localized discomfort it forces the body to compensate in order to maintain function. Here's how it happens:

- **Forward Head Posture:** A low or improperly functioning tongue can strain the deep front line, pulling the head forward and placing extra stress on the neck and shoulders.

- **Pelvic Tilt or Hip Imbalance:** Restrictions higher in the chain can cause compensatory tilts in the pelvis, leading to uneven gait or knee pain.

- **Foot and Ankle Issues:** Even the feet can bear the brunt of fascial imbalances originating from the head, affecting stability and alignment.

- **Diaphragmatic Dysfunction:** Tight fascia around the tongue and jaw impacts the deep front line, limiting diaphragm movement and restricting optimal breathing.

The Tongue as a Key Player

Your tongue is uniquely positioned at the top of the deep front line and acts as a "rudder" for posture and balance. When it's properly positioned on the roof of the mouth, it:

- Supports the natural curve of the spine.
- Reduces strain on the neck, jaw, and shoulders.
- Enhances breathing efficiency by stabilizing the airway.

On the flip side, a low tongue posture, tongue-tie, or jaw tension can disrupt this balance, leading to compensatory patterns that ripple through the entire fascial network.

The Meridian Connection: How Your Teeth Link to Your Body

Did you know that each tooth in your mouth is connected to an organ or system in your body through energy pathways called **meridians?** This concept comes from Traditional Chinese Medicine, which views the body as an interconnected system where disruptions in one area can affect another.

What Are Meridians?

Meridians are like energy highways running throughout your body, connecting different organs, tissues, and even your teeth. Each tooth is associated with a specific meridian, and problems with that tooth can reflect or contribute to imbalances in the related organ or body system.

For example:

- Your **upper central incisors** are connected to the kidney and bladder meridians.
- The **canines** are linked to the liver and gallbladder.
- The **molars** correspond to the stomach and spleen.

How Teeth Reflect Systemic Health

When there's an issue with a tooth such as decay, infection, or even a poorly placed filling it can disrupt the energy flow along the meridian, potentially contributing to problems in the associated organ or system. On the flip side, systemic issues can sometimes show up as sensitivity, pain, or inflammation in the corresponding teeth.

For instance:

- Chronic digestive issues might correlate with problems in your molars (stomach/spleen meridian).
- Hormonal imbalances can sometimes manifest in the premolars (reproductive organ meridian).
- Sinus congestion may be felt in the upper molars (linked to sinus and lung meridians).

Practical Implications

Understanding these connections gives us a more holistic view of health:

1. **When to Look Deeper:** If a specific tooth is persistently problematic, it might be worth investigating the health of the associated organ system.
2. **Partnering with Your Dentist and Doctor:** Collaboration between dental and medical professionals can help uncover hidden health issues.
3. **Supporting Whole-Body Wellness:** Maintaining good oral health including routine dental care, proper oral hygiene, and a balanced diet supports the health of your teeth and the systems they connect to.

What You Can Do

If you're curious about your own teeth-meridian connections, here are a few steps to get started:

- **Meridian Charts:** Many holistic dentists and practitioners use meridian charts that map the connection between teeth and organs. These can be a valuable tool for identifying potential links.
- **Work with a Holistic Dentist:** Dentists who take a whole-body approach can help you explore these connections and provide treatment that considers your overall health.
- **Address Oral and Systemic Health Together:** Don't ignore oral health problems, as they could be the key to resolving broader health issues.

The Bigger Picture

The connection between your teeth and your body's meridians is yet another way oral health ties into whole-body wellness. By caring for your teeth and being mindful of these connections, you're not just protecting your smile, you're supporting your entire system.

Restoring Balance: The Myofunctional Approach

By addressing oral posture and breathing with myofunctional therapy, we can help release tight fascia and restore balance across the entire body. Exercises that retrain the tongue, strengthen the jaw, and promote nasal breathing not only optimize oral function but also help realign the myofascial meridians.

Why It Matters:

Treating tight fascia isn't just about relieving a sore neck or improving posture. It's about recognizing that every restriction has a ripple effect. By targeting root causes like tongue posture and breathing, you unlock the potential for better alignment, improved mobility, and whole-body health.

The Importance of Myofunctional Therapy

Oral Myofunctional Therapy (OMT) uses targeted exercises to retrain the tongue and surrounding muscles, improving functions like swallowing, breathing, and speaking.

When paired with other treatments, such as tongue-tie releases or orthodontic care, myofunctional therapy helps create lasting improvements. No tongue should be released without a full evaluation and exercise after to prevent it from reattaching or blocking the airway due to lack of control.

Your tongue's position and function have far-reaching effects on your health, from breathing and sleep to posture and dental alignment. Correcting improper tongue positioning may feel overwhelming, but small, intentional steps—like becoming aware of your oral posture—can lead to significant improvements.

If you suspect a problem, consult a qualified professional. Remember, the journey to better health often begins with a single, well-informed choice.

Muscles Move Teeth or hold them in place

The muscles of your tongue, mouth and face are nature's orthodontic stabilizers. They can have an influence on the movement and position of our teeth.

Teeth are ever-changing, they can be altered and moved by muscular influence from the jaws, lips, cheeks and tongue. This is why early intervention is important because: **Form Follows function.**

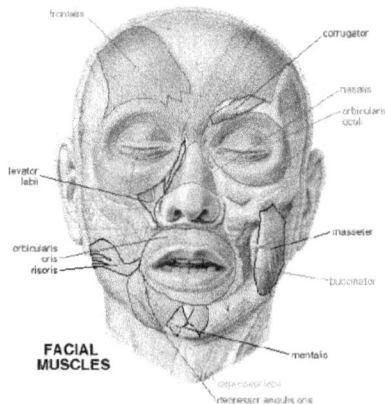

FACIAL MUSCLES

The same forces used by wearing braces can also be used by the tongue to move teeth. We swallow 800- 2000 times per day. If your tongue pushes forward, it is putting 1 pound of pressure against the teeth every time you swallow. You can see how if not corrected your teeth will keep moving.

The shape of the face changes along with the position of the teeth.

Ideally, a balance of forces exists between the lips and cheeks on the outside of the teeth, and the tongue on the inside of the teeth. Any imbalances affect the growth, comfort, and position of the teeth and jaw.

The most significant type of muscular imbalance to affect the oral and facial structures is called a "tongue thrust" or "reverse swallow."

If you have braces, and a untreated tongue thrust it can be a problem because:

- It can slow down your orthodontic treatment, keeping your braces on for a longer time.
- It can make your teeth move again, after your braces are taken off.
- It can make moving your teeth and closing spaces much more difficult for your orthodontist. When the muscles of your mouth and face are not in balance, solving orthodontic problems is much more challenging.

How do you know if you have a tongue thrust?

There are many characteristics to look for in order to determine if you, or your child, have a tongue thrust.

Below are 4 of the most common signs to recognize:

1. **Mouth breathing** is the most common sign. The mouth is open at rest, and the tongue is often forward or sticking out.
2. **Speech Concerns**, especially lisping, can be a sign of a tongue thrust. If there is difficulty pronouncing "T, D, N, and L" sounds, this is another indicator. General problems with articulation, rate of speech, and voice quality and clarity may also be present.
3. **Sucking habits**, past or present, can cause a tongue thrust to develop. The formation of the mouth and position of the tongue are changed by the thumb or finger during a sucking habit. Even if the child quits

the habit, the damage caused to the function of the tongue, facial musculature, and other structures often still remains.

4. **Open Bite** having front or side teeth unable to bite together is an excellent sign of a swallowing dysfunction.

How do you treat a tongue thrust swallow?

Treating a tongue thrust swallow typically involves retraining the tongue to move in the correct swallowing pattern, through exercises and therapy, which involves pushing up and back against the roof of the mouth instead of pushing forward against the front teeth.

In severe cases, orthodontic treatment may be necessary to correct any dental problems caused by the tongue thrust swallow.

Treatment may include:

1. Tongue exercises: A speech-language pathologist or an orofacial myologist can teach you exercises to strengthen the tongue and retrain it to move in the correct swallowing pattern.
2. Myofunctional therapy: This type of therapy focuses on retraining the muscles of the face, tongue, and mouth to correct the swallowing pattern.
3. Orthodontic treatment: In some cases, orthodontic treatment may be necessary to correct any dental problems caused by the tongue thrust swallow, such as misaligned teeth or an open bite.
4. Behavior modification: Making certain changes to your daily habits can also help correct a tongue thrust swallow. For example, avoiding sucking on straws, chewing gum, or biting your nails can help prevent the tongue from pushing forward against the teeth.
5. Counseling: Counseling may be necessary if a tongue thrust swallow is related to an underlying emotional or behavioral issue.

What can happen if you do not have treatment for a tongue thrust swallow

If a tongue thrust swallow is not treated, it can lead to several potential complications, including:

1. Dental problems: The repeated pushing of the tongue against the front teeth can cause misalignment of the teeth, leading to issues such as an open bite, overbite, or other orthodontic problems.
2. Speech difficulties: A tongue thrust swallow can interfere with normal speech patterns, causing speech difficulties such as lisping or difficulty pronouncing certain sounds.
3. Swallowing difficulties: A tongue thrust swallow can also lead to difficulty swallowing, particularly with larger pieces of food.
4. Choking: In severe cases, a tongue thrust swallow can lead to choking, particularly when eating or drinking.
5. Self-esteem issues: Dental and speech problems caused by a tongue thrust swallow can lead to self-esteem issues, particularly in children and adolescents.

It is important to seek the advice of a qualified healthcare professional, such as a speech-language pathologist, dentist, or orthodontist, to determine the best course of treatment for a tongue thrust swallow to prevent these potential complications.

Who can treat a tongue thrust swallow?

A tongue thrust swallow can be treated by several healthcare professionals, including:

1. Speech-Language Pathologist: A speech-language pathologist (SLP) is a healthcare professional who specializes in evaluating and treating communication disorders, including tongue thrust swallow. SLPs can provide exercises and therapy to retrain the tongue to move in the correct swallowing pattern.
2. Orofacial Myologist: An orofacial myologist (also known as myofunctional therapist) is a healthcare professional who specializes in the treatment of oral and facial muscles. They can provide therapy to retrain the tongue and other oral muscles to correct the swallowing pattern.
3. Dentist: A dentist can evaluate the teeth and oral structures for any damage or misalignment caused by a tongue thrust swallow. They can also provide orthodontic treatment if necessary to correct any dental problems.

4. Orthodontist: An orthodontist is a specialist in the diagnosis, prevention, and treatment of dental and facial irregularities. They can provide orthodontic treatment to correct any dental problems caused by a tongue thrust swallow.

5. Pediatrician: A pediatrician can evaluate children for a tongue thrust swallow and refer them to a speech-language pathologist or other specialist for further evaluation and treatment.

Orthodontists have struggled over the years, fighting the strength of the tongue while trying to provide the best orthodontic treatment. Years ago orthodontists would install barbaric looking appliances to try to curb a tongue habit. Who am I kidding, some still do.

Today many orthodontists refer to myofunctional therapists to treat tongue thrust swallowing. We first assess the underlying causes of the tongue thrust swallow such as tongue tie, tongue space, oral habits, airway or breathing problems. Once underlying causes of the tongue thrust swallow are addressed your therapist will teach correct tongue posture and correct swallowing patterns which are then habituated into your daily life.

Oral Myofunctional Therapy is another method used for eliminating a tongue thrust. It is an exercise-based treatment that teaches patients how to use their tongue and facial muscles normally. We touched on this earlier.

An Oral Myofunctional Therapist (OMT) can be an instrumental figure in helping a patient learn to retrain the facial muscles and eliminate a tongue thrusting habit. OMTs are skilled at helping children and adults gain control over muscular habits, including those involved in a tongue thrust. For children and adults who struggle with tongue thrusting, stopping the habit is not always easy. This is because all of the muscles of the face and mouth have been programmed over the course of many years. The person's body does not know how to use the tongue and facial muscles correctly, and needs help.

A consultation with an oral myofunctional therapist can be very valuable. If the muscles are not re-trained, your orthodontic treatment and final result may be compromised.

Besides affecting your braces, a tongue thrust can also have a lasting negative impact on a person's general health, speech, dental health, swallowing and breathing throughout life.

If your tongue is not resting correctly in your mouth due to a jaw issue or tongue-tie, things can get out of alignment in your mouth and the rest of your body.

What is a posterior tongue tie?

A posterior tongue-tie is a restriction of the fascia and a relatively new concept to many people in the dental field but I'm seeing a lot of patients with posterior tongue-ties in my practice, so I thought I'd go into some detail about this condition. We were only taught to look for an anterior tongue tie and that it was only a problem if an infant could not latch, could not stick out the tongue or started to have a speech issue.

Anterior tongue-ties are obvious. This is the kind of tongue-tie that's most easily diagnosed and treated. We can see right away that the underside of the tongue is connected too tightly to the floor of the mouth, and that the range of motion is restricted.

A tongue-tie, also known as ankyloglossia, is a condition that develops in babies in utero and is present at birth. Tongue-ties restrict the movement of the tongue and limit its range of motion in the mouth. There are two types: anterior and posterior. However we are getting away from this classification as we learn more.

We've been hearing a lot about tongue-ties lately as modern medicine starts to recognize the negative health effects of a tongue-tie and restrictions. The tongue is connected through our facia system all the way to our toes. Kids that walk on their toes may have tight fascia or a restriction.

Tongue-ties can negatively impact a baby's ability to eat and swallow. Other consequences of a tongue-tie for infants include:

- Difficulty breastfeeding, often resulting in early termination of breastfeeding
- Negative impacts on milk supply

- Diagnosis of failure to thrive
- Poor sleep
- Difficulty adjusting to solid foods

Children with tongue-ties also experience issues such as:

- Difficulty eating solid foods
- Gagging or choking
- Unwillingness to try new foods; only eating certain foods
- Drooling
- Aversion to certain foods
- Speech delay or speech issues like deterioration in speech or difficulty articulating
- Behavior problems, including ADD/ADHD, ODD, depression and mood swings
- Dental issues such as crowded teeth
- Behaviors to compensate for tongue-tie that may be hard to break

And, if these issues remain untreated into adulthood, other issues can develop. These issues can directly impact how you feel about yourself, how you relate or interact with others, and your dental and overall health.

Adults with tongue-ties frequently experience issues including:

- The inability to open the mouth and restricted tongue movement that widely affects speech and eating habits
- Speech impediments; stress over having to focus on speaking properly
- An inability to speak clearly
- Noisy jaw joints (creaking, clicking, grating or popping of the jaw)
- Pain in the jaws at rest or when in use
- Headaches
- Jaw development issues
- Poor oral health, including tooth decay and gingivitis
- Stress or sensitivity about appearance

Tongue-ties can also affect your posture. If there is a tongue-tie present, the head tends to be tilted low and forward.

Forward head posture related to tongue-tie can also stress the sternocleidomastoid muscle (SCM) and the trapezius muscle, as well as muscles in the back and neck, and contribute to:

- Jaw conditions, such as TMD
- Neck and back pain
- Headaches/migraines
- Pain in the shoulder

Tongue-ties can also affect your breathing (causing mouth breathing), the stability of your pelvic floor and even how you walk.

If you notice these effects in yourself or your child, it is time to talk about treating that tongue-tie. While you may think it's relatively harmless, the fact is that this condition can affect the entire body and overall health.

Tongue-ties and complications are treated with myofunctional therapy and surgery to release restricted tissue. Many individuals treated for their tongue-tie find immediate relief from their symptoms, including improved posture.

Not everyone with a tongue tie should have a release! It depends on the severity, symptoms, and function. Is there enough room for your tongue? Do you have hypermobility syndrome, Ehlers-Danlos syndrome or retained primitive reflexes?

Recommendation: Your child will not outgrow many of these issues. It is important to seek the advice of a qualified healthcare professional to determine the best course of treatment for a tongue thrust swallow and tongue ties. Not all ties should be released with surgery. For some, releasing could make breathing more difficult or cause other issues.

Real-Life Benefits of Myofunctional Therapy

Let me share a quick example: A child I worked with struggled with mouth breathing and frequent headaches. Through myofunctional therapy, we trained their tongue to rest on the roof of their mouth, encouraged nasal breathing, and improved their swallowing technique. The results? Better sleep, reduced headaches, and a happier kid!

Another client, an adult with TMJ pain, found relief just by addressing oral posture and jaw alignment through simple exercises. No fancy tools, just targeted, consistent practice.

What You Can Do Today

Here's how you can get started:

1. **Check Your Tongue Posture:** Is your tongue resting on the roof of your mouth? If not, practice gently placing it there.
2. **Breathe Through Your Nose:** Consciously switch to nasal breathing throughout the day.
3. **Close Your Lips:** Keep your lips gently sealed when you're at rest, letting your tongue and nasal breathing do their jobs.

Finding Support: Posture Therapy and Chiropractic Care

When it comes to improving posture and restoring alignment, there are professionals and resources that can help guide you. While myofunctional therapy focuses on the head and neck, addressing posture often requires a team approach. Here's where you can look for support:

1. Chiropractors

Chiropractors specialize in spinal alignment and can help identify and address imbalances caused by poor posture. They often use adjustments and exercises to restore proper alignment, relieve pain, and improve mobility.

How to find one:

- Look for chiropractors with a focus on posture correction or functional movement.
- Ask if they incorporate lifestyle advice and exercises for long-term posture improvement.

2. Posture Restoration Therapists

Postural restoration therapy focuses on retraining your body to use the correct muscles for balance and alignment. This approach can be particularly helpful for chronic pain or compensatory patterns.

Where to start:

- Search for therapists certified by organizations like the Postural Restoration Institute (PRI).
- Look for professionals who offer a combination of assessments, exercises, and tailored treatment plans.

3. Physical Therapists

A physical therapist can provide exercises to strengthen weak muscles, release tight areas, and improve posture. They often collaborate with other specialists to create a comprehensive plan.

Tips for finding one:

- Seek out physical therapists who specialize in postural rehabilitation or chronic pain management.
- Many PTs incorporate myofascial release or targeted stretching into their therapy.

4. Yoga and Pilates Instructors

Yoga and Pilates can help improve posture, flexibility, and core strength, all of which support overall alignment. Many instructors are trained to recognize and address postural issues through movement and mindful breathing.

Getting started:

- Look for instructors certified in therapeutic yoga or Pilates.
- Consider classes focused on posture and alignment, such as restorative yoga or reformer Pilates.

5. Online Resources and Tools

If you're not ready to see a professional in person, there are plenty of online resources to help you get started:

- **Apps and Platforms:** Posture apps like UPRIGHT GO or online programs like Foundation Training.
- **Books and Videos:** Look for resources from experts in posture restoration or movement therapy.

- **Workshops and Webinars:** Many practitioners offer virtual events to teach posture correction techniques.

How Myofunctional Therapy Fits In

While these professionals address body-wide posture, myofunctional therapy focuses specifically on the head and neck. Combining myofunctional therapy with posture support can help you tackle alignment from top to bottom.

Myofunctional therapy may be needed to retrain their tongue and orofacial muscles before and after their tongue-tie is treated, for tongue thrust swallow or other issues.

Learn more about our service go to my website www.shereewertz.com or schedule a free consultation to chat. If I can not help you I will find you someone who can.

Ehlers-Danlos Syndrome

The Ehlers-Danlos syndromes (EDS) are a group of 13 heritable connective tissue disorders. The conditions are caused by genetic changes that affect connective tissue. Each type of EDS has its own set of features.

Some features associated with EDS, include joint hypermobility, skin hyperextensibility, and tissue fragility.

Signs and symptoms of EDS range greatly based on the type of syndrome you have—different types impact different areas of the body. For example, some people with EDS are most affected in their eyes or teeth, but the hypermobile type causes musculoskeletal and joint problems.

While hypermobile EDS is the most common type, it is also the least severe. Symptoms can vary greatly: Some people with hypermobile EDS have mildly loose or very flexible joints, but others experience chronic pain from joint dislocation. Infants and toddlers who have hypermobile EDS have weaker muscles, which means motor milestones like sitting, standing, or walking may occur later than babies without EDS.

Tongue ties in people with forms of EDS should be evaluated as a release may make things much worse or not heal as anticipated. I am very cautious in recomming a release to someone with this syndrome.

There is no cure for EDS, but that doesn't mean that you can't enjoy a full and happy life. Talk to your medical team about prevention strategies and therapies that may help stabilize your joints, reduce pain, and increase your quality of life.

What is the prevalence of EDS?

Each type of EDS has a different prevalence in the population. Hypermobile EDS (hEDS) is the most common type of EDS by far. hEDS accounts for about 90% of EDS cases and is thought to affect at least 1 in 3,100-5,000 people.

What causes EDS?

EDS is caused by specific variants in genes that provide the instructions for making collagens and related connective tissue proteins. Some types of EDS are associated with multiple different genes.

Many people with a type of Ehlers-Danlos syndrome (EDS) or hypermobility spectrum disorder (HSD) experience issues with:

- Sleep initiation (falling asleep)
- Sleep maintenance (staying asleep)
- Sleep restoration (getting refreshing sleep)

There are many reasons a person with a type of EDS or HSD may have sleeping issues. Management of sleeping issues should focus on their underlying cause(s).

There is not a lot of discussion about EDS and it is often missed or not even looked at.

https://www.healthcentral.com/condition/sacroiliac-joint-pain/ehlers-danlos-syndrome-sacroiliac-joint-dysfunction

FAQ

Does insurance cover therapy?

The coverage of tongue thrust therapy by insurance may vary depending on the individual insurance plan and the provider's diagnosis. In general, speech therapy for speech and language disorders is often covered by insurance, including treatment for tongue thrust. However, it is important to check with your specific insurance provider to confirm coverage for tongue thrust therapy.

It may also be helpful to check with the speech-language pathologist or orofacial myologist who will be providing the therapy to see if they accept your insurance and if they can provide information about the insurance coverage for tongue thrust therapy.

If insurance does not cover tongue thrust therapy, there may be other options for financial assistance, such as government-funded programs, grants, or payment plans offered by the healthcare provider.

Tongue Health

Your tongue is something you need to look at consistently. Have you ever really looked at your tongue?

Open your mouth and look at your tongue. That may sound strange, but your tongue can tell a lot about your health. If your tongue is bright red like a strawberry, it could be a sign of a deficiency in folic acid, vitamin B12, or iron.

A black and hairy looking tongue can signal poor oral hygiene.

OK, if your tongue is blue, it's likely from that blue ring pop you just ate or a mouth rinse you used. Other colors, however, could signal certain health issues. While many tongue color changes are harmless, some could be a sign of something worthy of having it checked out by your doctor.

Here's what your tongue color could be telling you about your health.

Swollen tongue

If your tongue is larger than normal it could be an indication of several things. You will need to figure out just what it means.

It could be as simple as you ate something spicy that made it swell.

You are having an allergic reaction to something.

A swollen tongue is one sign of hypothyroidism.

Dehydration may be indicated by a swollen or scalloped tongue.

If you are not sure what the cause is, or it persists, follow up with a checkup, this is not normal. Only you know how it feels if you have cause for concern, follow up.

White tongue

If your tongue is white, it could again be something you ate, or it could mean there's a buildup of bacteria, debris, and cells on your papillae (those bumps on your tongue that contain taste buds). It's usually harmless and can be removed by brushing and/or scraping your tongue.

If your tongue is white with red (sometimes bleeding) bumps, it could mean you have a fungal infection called oral thrush. Oral thrush is caused by types of yeast fungus called Candida that live in your mouth.

It's not usually painful, but it can give your mouth an unpleasant cottony or burning feeling that can make it hard to eat, speak and, with severe infections, hard to swallow. If left untreated it can last for months or years, it's rarely dangerous, but it can move into the bloodstream and cause life-threatening blood poisoning. Thrush is typically treated with antifungal medications.

Red tongue

If your tongue is swollen and bright red, it could be inflamed from a vitamin B12 deficiency.

Vitamin B12 deficiency is a low red blood cell count due to a lack of the vitamin B12, which can cause a swollen, red tongue. It can look like your teeth are imprinted in your tongue. You could also have cracks in the corners of your mouth known as angular cheilitis.

Black Hairy Tongue

It is ugly, yet temporary and harmless. Black hairy tongue seems to be more common in men.

Black hairy tongue is happening because there is an overgrowth of bacteria and dead sloughing cells that build up on the tiny rounded projections on the tongue called papillae. Normally the papilla are pinkish-white.

Certain types of bacteria accumulate on your tongue, that stain the papillae and make the tongue look different colors most commonly black or brown. But I have seen yellow and green also.

If normal shedding of the cells on the tongue become inhibited, they grow and lengthen creating hair like projections which make the tongue appear hairy. They can grow up to 15 times their normal length.

Causes of Black Hairy Tongue

Black hairy tongue is caused by too much bacteria in the mouth, by a reduced saliva flow in your mouth or from things like smoking, food, drinking coffee and tea, yeast, mouth breathing, poor diet, illness, medications, chewing tobacco, use of alcohol and poor oral hygiene.

Certain conditions that disrupt the normal balance of bacteria in your mouth can make you more likely to develop a black hairy tongue.

Here are a few:

Undergoing cancer treatments
Use of Antibiotics
Dry mouth
Being dehydrated
HIV
IV drug use

Symptoms of Black Hairy Tongue

Most people don't even know they have a black hairy tongue unless they look at their tongue and there are no symptoms or discomfort.

Some people report they have a metallic taste due to the presence of the thickening of the papillae.

Others have reported a tickling feeling. If the papillae grow extra-long in severe cases it may lead to bad breath or a gagging feeling.

Treatment for white or black hairy tongue

Brush

Black hairy tongue can be resolved simply by gently brushing your tongue twice a day as part of your daily dental routine.

Use a tongue scraper.

Drink plenty of water.

Maintain good oral hygiene and regular visits to the dentist.

Other than the appearance of the tongue most people don't even know they have it.

Rinse

Brush or swish with 1-part hydrogen peroxide and 5 parts water, then rinse with plain water.

Do not rinse with straight hydrogen peroxide daily or for longer than 5 minutes.

If you have essential oils, you can also add tea tree or peppermint oil to the mixture.

Avoid mouth rinses that contain alcohol or witch hazel.

If it persists, see your dental professional or your physician.

If the condition does not get better on its own with brushing and tongue scraping, they can prescribe a medication or use the laser to remove the papillae.

Like everything in your mouth, if you take care and brush your tongue regularly you can prevent most of these situations from occurring.

The Oral-Systemic Connection

Many systemic diseases first present themselves with symptoms in the mouth. A patient undergoing open-heart surgery, for instance, is now required to get a dental clearance to ensure their mouth is free of infection before the operation. Why? Because we know that the health of the mouth can have life-altering consequences for the rest of the body.

Just as the blood-brain barrier protects the brain from toxins in the blood, there's a barrier that shields our bloodstream from the bacteria in our mouths. Gum disease, however, can compromise this barrier, allowing bacteria and inflammation to travel beyond the oral cavity and contribute to systemic diseases.

The Role of Inflammation

Inflammation is believed to be a major factor in the oral-systemic link. Chronic inflammation in the gums, such as from periodontal disease, doesn't remain confined to the mouth. It creates a ripple effect, influencing other inflammatory conditions throughout the body. Treating gum inflammation can often alleviate symptoms or improve outcomes for conditions like diabetes, heart disease, and more.

Diseases Strongly Linked to Oral Health

Cancer

Research from the American Academy of Periodontology indicates a troubling connection between gum disease and certain cancers:

- Pancreatic cancer: **54% increased risk**
- Kidney cancer: **49% increased risk**
- Blood cancers: **30% increased risk**

Respiratory Disease

Bacteria from the mouth can be inhaled into the lungs, causing respiratory infections like pneumonia. Aspiration pneumonia, particularly common in nursing home patients, often stems from poor oral care.

Heart Disease and Stroke

Chronic inflammation from gum disease is linked to an increased risk of cardiovascular diseases, including heart attacks and strokes.

Diabetes

There's a two-way relationship between diabetes and gum disease:

- Diabetes worsens gum disease by impairing blood flow and immune response.

- Gum disease makes blood sugar levels harder to control. Addressing one often improves the other.

Other Conditions Linked to Oral Health

- **Irritable bowel syndrome (IBS)**
- **Breast and prostate cancer**
- **Dementia and Alzheimer's disease**
- **Osteoporosis**
- **Rheumatoid arthritis**
- **Pregnancy complications** (e.g., preterm birth and low birth weight)
- **Weight gain and obesity**
- **Kidney disease**

Why Early Action Matters

The evidence is clear: oral health impacts far more than just your teeth and gums. Ignoring signs like bleeding gums, bad breath, or persistent inflammation can allow systemic diseases to go undetected.

Much like my own experience with bleeding gums alerting me to cancer, these early oral symptoms can act as warning signs for bigger issues. Addressing them promptly isn't just about preserving your smile, it could save your life.

Taking Control of Your Oral and Overall Health

Preventing and treating gum disease is crucial for maintaining overall health. Here are some steps you can take to protect both your mouth and body:

1. **Practice Consistent Oral Hygiene:** Brush twice a day, floss regularly, and clean your tongue to reduce bacteria.
2. **Seek Dental Care Proactively:** Visit your dentist at least twice a year, and don't hesitate to ask questions about your overall health.
3. **Pay Attention to Symptoms:** Bleeding gums, bad breath, and sensitivity can indicate larger health issues.
4. **Adopt an Anti-Inflammatory Lifestyle:** Maintain a healthy diet, exercise regularly, and get enough sleep.
5. **Communicate With Healthcare Providers:** Advocate for oral health discussions as part of your medical treatment plan.

The more we learn about the relationship between oral health and systemic conditions, the more apparent it becomes that we can no longer afford to treat the mouth separately from the body. Be your own advocate for healthcare.

How Does the Mouth Affect the Body?

Your mouth is a bustling ecosystem of bacteria. Plaque and bacteria continuously build up on your teeth. If left undisturbed, this bacteria multiplies, feeding on sugars from the food and drinks you consume. This creates acid, which can weaken your teeth and gums, making them more susceptible to infection.

The mouth is not just the gateway to the body, it's often the first line of defense. Let's treat it that way. The mouth is not just where digestion begins; it is a critical gateway to your overall health. What happens in your mouth doesn't stay there; it has ripple effects on the rest of your body. To truly understand how your mouth impacts your health, let's start with what's happening in your oral cavity.

When the immune system steps in to combat these infections, it causes inflammation, a natural response that, if prolonged, can have serious consequences. Chronic inflammation in the mouth doesn't just affect the gums and teeth. It can break down the barrier that normally protects the bloodstream, allowing bacteria to travel throughout the body and contribute to systemic conditions.

The Progression of Dental Disease

Dental disease typically follows a predictable pattern:

1. Cavities: Often overlooked as minor, cavities are the result of bacteria-produced acid eroding tooth enamel. Cavities are the #1 preventable childhood disease, in fact and are completely reversible in the early stages.
2. Gingivitis: This inflammation of the gums is an early warning sign that your mouth is under attack. It is also 100% reversible if addressed promptly.
3. Periodontitis: Left untreated, gingivitis progresses to gum disease, or periodontitis. In this advanced stage, inflammation causes gums to pull away from the teeth, creating pockets that trap more bacteria and food debris. Over time, this leads to bone loss, abscesses, and eventually tooth loss.
4. Systemic Impact: Chronic gum inflammation can allow bacteria and toxins to enter the bloodstream, triggering widespread inflammation in the body. This adds stress to your immune system, forcing it to fight on multiple fronts.

The Silent Threat of Dental Infections

One of the biggest dangers of dental infections is their stealth. In many cases, you won't feel pain or notice a problem until the infection has advanced. By this stage, bacteria may already be spreading to other parts of the body, potentially causing complications like:

- Facial swelling or abscesses
- Bloodstream infections (sepsis)
- Heart infections (endocarditis)
- Liver or kidney infections

If you experience symptoms such as bleeding gums, toothaches, fever, or jaw pain, it's crucial to seek treatment immediately.

Prevention: Your First Line of Defense

The good news? You have the power to prevent most oral health problems with consistent habits and informed choices.

Actionable Steps for Oral Health:

1. Brush Twice Daily: Use a fluoride toothpaste and a soft-bristled brush to clean teeth and gums. Spend at least two minutes brushing each time.
2. Floss or Use a Water Flosser: Clean between teeth daily to remove plaque and debris where your toothbrush can't reach.
3. Breathe Through Your Nose: Mouth breathing dries out oral tissues, increasing the risk of gum disease and cavities.
4. Hydrate: Drinking water helps wash away food particles and maintains healthy saliva production.
5. Eat an Anti-Inflammatory Diet: Choose nutrient-rich, low-sugar foods to support both oral and systemic health.
6. Monitor Signs of Gum Disease: Bleeding gums, persistent bad breath, and gum recession are early warnings to take seriously.
7. See Your Dentist Regularly: Professional cleanings and checkups can catch issues before they become major problems.

Breaking the Cycle of Avoidance

Many patients avoid the dentist out of fear, embarrassment, or financial concerns. They wait until pain becomes unbearable, often requiring more extensive (and expensive) treatment.

Remember, dentistry is preventive care. Just as routine oil changes keep your car running smoothly, regular dental visits maintain the health of your mouth and body.

Cavities and Gum Disease: The Silent Threat

What Are Cavities?

Cavities, also known as tooth decay, are permanently damaged areas in the enamel. They are caused by harmful bacteria that feed on sugars and starches, producing acid that erodes the hard surface of the teeth.

What Are Gum Disease and Its Stages?

Gum disease begins with **gingivitis**, marked by red, swollen gums that bleed when brushed or flossed. Without intervention, it progresses to **periodontitis**, where the gums pull away from the teeth, forming deep pockets that harbor bacteria.

If untreated, periodontitis can lead to:

- **Tooth loss**
- **Bone loss**
- **Systemic inflammation** affecting the heart, lungs, and more

The Domino Effect: How Oral Health Impacts the Body

Think of your mouth as the front line of your body's health. Chronic inflammation caused by gum disease or untreated cavities doesn't stay confined to your mouth. Bacteria can enter your bloodstream, traveling to other organs and increasing your risk for:

- **Heart disease and stroke**: Inflammation from oral infections can damage blood vessels.
- **Diabetes**: Gum disease worsens blood sugar control.
- **Cancer**: Studies have shown links between periodontal disease and cancers like pancreatic, kidney, and blood cancers.
- **Respiratory issues**: Bacteria from the mouth can be inhaled, causing infections like pneumonia.

At any given time, your mouth is full of bacteria. Some of this bacteria is beneficial and helps you digest food, while other bacteria can be harmful. The harmful bacteria feeds on the sugar and starch in the food you eat. As the bacteria feed they produce an acid. Over time, that acid weakens the surface of the teeth and begins to create a hole in your enamel, otherwise known as a cavity. It is important to address cavities as quickly as possible.

Although there are other factors that can make you more likely to get cavities, they are almost 100% preventable with the right diet, proper home care, nasal breathing and controlling the pH levels of your mouth! The American Academy of Pediatric Dentistry (AAPD) states that 60 percent of children will have a cavity by the age of 5. I saw this when I was working in a mobile setting. We can change these statistics together.

Can a cavity heal or go away?

Some experts say enamel on the surface of a tooth can get some of its minerals back with fluoride, calcium phosphate and hydroxyapatite. You can slow decay down and maybe even stop it when it is on the enamel surface. Called incipient decay.

Tooth decay can be stopped or reversed at this point. Enamel can repair itself by using minerals from saliva, calcium phosphate, hydroxyapatite, and fluoride from toothpaste or other sources or products that remineralize. But if the tooth decay process continues, more minerals are lost, the bacteria and decay get through that enamel, and reach the inner layer called Dentin, the damage is done. Cavities won't go away on their own, the cavity is permanent damage that will require a dentist to repair the tooth and fill the hole.

How serious is a cavity?

If cavities aren't treated, they get larger and deeper into the dentin layer of your teeth. If left untreated they can lead to a severe toothache, infection, tooth loss and possible health issues. If it goes untreated to that point you may need to have the tooth removed.

The decay will spread, both outwards across the enamel and deeper inside towards the root of the tooth. If it reaches the root or nerve of the tooth the tooth will require a root canal to save it. The bacteria that cause decay can also spread to other family members through kissing, sharing utensils, drinks and straws.

How do we treat decay?

When you have a hole in your tooth that is full of acid-producing bacteria working to make the hole even bigger. It is the dentist's job to remove the damaged tooth structure and to put a filling in to replace the part of the tooth that was damaged.

A filling is like a puzzle piece that the dentist shapes to fit the hole in your tooth. Sometimes, the damage to your tooth can be so bad that the bacteria can reach the inner layer of your tooth, the nerve and blood vessels also called "pulp", and cause severe pain and infection. In this case, your tooth can be saved with a root canal, which is a procedure where the affected nerve is removed from your tooth in order to get you out of pain and to prevent you from losing your tooth. The tooth has now lost its nutrient supply making it brittle. Your dentist will recommend a crown to protect that tooth so it can handle the chewing forces preventing it from breaking in the future.

However, if the tooth decay is too large the dentist may not be able to save your tooth and it may need to be extracted.

Many people opt to just have the tooth removed because it is cheaper to just take it out. The cost can be over $5000 to save it and repair the damage with a root canal and a crown.

However what is not always discussed is what happens once you lose a tooth. Now you have a big space which can affect your ability to chew. This has an effect on your digestion, you may not be able to chew as long or effectively so now your stomach has to take up the slack breaking down bigger pieces of food or you only chew on one side. When you chew on one side you develop the muscles uneven on one side of your face. One eye or eyebrow may be higher than the other. When you smile it is uneven and so on. If the tooth above or below that space does not have an opposing tooth it will keep growing causing the other teeth to shift creating traumatic occlusion or putting more forces on other teeth. I hope you can see the domino effect that can be created.

How can I prevent cavities?

With good home care, brushing, flossing, waterpik, a healthy balanced diet, controlling the pH and acid will help minimize your risk for decay and help you keep your teeth for a lifetime.

It is important to know that even though you may have had your teeth "fixed" by your dentist in the past, you can get a new cavity around a filling easier than in a healthy tooth. Even though it is the dentist's job to help fix your teeth, it is still just as important for you to take good care of the work they have done with daily habits.

What does bleeding in the mouth mean?

Bleeding gums are usually caused by inadequate plaque removal. Which means you are not brushing enough, or you are missing areas in your mouth.

Plaque contains bacteria that attack the healthy tissue around the teeth. Which in turn cause the gums to become inflamed, irritated, and bleed when brushing or flossing. This is called gingivitis and is the first stage of gum disease.

Gingivitis

One out of two people in the United States has Gingivitis right now as I write this book!

If you follow me, you heard me state this repeatedly.

Almost everyone has had gingivitis at some point in their life. You can have it on just one tooth or in just one area of the mouth. You may not even know you have it or have had it. I see people every day that do not know they have it.

You can see there are many reasons your gums may be inflamed or swollen. Whatever the reason, if you catch it early enough, you can change it by simply just taking the time to brush all the areas of your mouth.

Slowing down and massaging the gums with your toothbrush, removing the plaque and biofilm. Establishing a methodical tooth brushing routine will almost guarantee a healthy mouth and healthy gums.

For most people all you will need to do is brush your gums two times a day, an eclectic toothbrush is best. Which toothbrush you use is really a personal preference. The tool you choose to use is not as important as how you use it. Some people do just fine with a manual brush. However, many do not.

After you brush your teeth, if you take your fingernail or toothpick and run it along your gums and see plaque, you did not remove it all, you will need to brush again or use floss or a water Flosser.

You can also use chewable disclosing tablets or a smart rinse that stains the plaque pink or blue to show you where you missed. Then brush again to get off the stained plaque.

What you do every day at home morning and night to take care of your teeth and gums is what is going to dictate if you have Gingivitis or cavities and how healthy your mouth will be for your life.

I have people every day tell me dentistry is expensive. My question is compared to what?

Most things in life are expensive these days. It is a matter of what you place value on.

Prevention is not expensive, fixing problems once they have gone past a certain point in any situation is expensive. Maintenance on your car or home is much easier to handle and pay for before a problem gets too big.

Fixing a leak in your roof is cheaper than doing nothing and waiting until there is a hole in your roof. The problem is much bigger and more expensive to fix.

Your mouth and teeth are the same. If you take steps to prevent and maintain them you most likely will not have problems in the future that seem too big and expensive to fix. No pain does not mean no problem.

It has been proven the health of your mouth not only affects your teeth, it also has a direct impact on the health of your body. Our body is great at making compensations to keep us alive, but if we do not give it what it needs it will break down.

We get warning signs that there is a problem and we ignore them until we can't.

Know Your Numbers

If you've visited a dentist, you may have heard numbers like 1–3 millimeters when your hygienist measures your gum pockets. Here's what they mean:

- 1–3 mm: Healthy gums with no bleeding
- 4–5 mm: Early signs of gum disease requiring deeper cleaning
- 6+ mm: Advanced periodontitis needing specialized care

Your numbers are your mouth's way of communicating its health status. Knowing them helps you stay proactive.

Your dental professional will use a periodontal probe to measure the depth of your gums in millimeters surrounding your teeth to find out how healthy your gums are.

When your hygienist is done with the measurements, they will explain their findings.

They can perform a cleaning if your gums are 1-3mm.

If you have a few fours with bleeding, and no bone loss is present you may need more than one cleaning.

Your first cleaning will be what we call a "prophy with inflammation."

If you have too much bleeding it is hard to see if we were able to remove all of the tartar and bacteria. When we are cleaning your teeth, we go by feel under the gum tissue, too much bleeding gives us a false smooth surface, or we can burnish the tarter on the root surface and not get it all off, doing you a disservice.

After the first cleaning we need to let you go home, brush the gums for a few weeks, reduce the gingivitis and bleeding and bring you back to make sure we have removed all the tartar and bacteria that can lead to periodontal disease in your mouth and other diseases in your body.

Your hygienist cannot do a normal cleaning if your measurements are greater than four. You may need to be numb, so we can perform what is called a deep cleaning (Scaling and root planing).

This is where we not only clean the teeth but also remove bacteria from the surrounding tissues. Some offices will use a laser for this procedure, reducing the bacteria in the pocket wall, allowing your body a chance to heal, decreasing the pocket depth so your toothbrush can do the job it is intended for.

What the numbers are telling you.

Your numbers can tell you:

Do you have a healthy mouth?

Do you have an active infection, if you have numbers over 4 mm they tell you what stage of disease you are in.

Do you have bleeding when probing? If yes it can mean an active infection.

Depending on findings, it lets the provider know what treatment to recommend.

> A more frequent care.
>
> A deeper cleaning.
>
> A visit to a specialist.

Gum Disease

According to the Centers for Disease Control and Prevention, half of adults age 30 and older suffer from some form of gum disease.

Periodontal disease and tooth decay are the two biggest threats to dental health.

Gum disease, an infection of the tissues that surround and support your teeth, is caused by plaque, the sticky film of bacteria that is constantly forming on our teeth. Plaque that is not removed with thorough daily brushing and cleaning between teeth can eventually harden into calculus or tartar. Periodontal disease and tooth decay are the two biggest threats to dental health.

There are four stages of gum disease; the earliest stage of gum disease is Gingivitis manifested by swollen, red gums and sometimes bad breath. Bleeding gums is one of the most common symptoms and the easiest to notice.

Stages 1-4

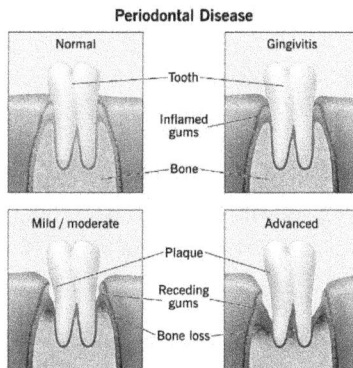

Periodontal Disease

Normal — Tooth, Inflamed gums, Bone

Gingivitis

Mild / moderate — Plaque, Receding gums, Bone loss

Advanced

Cleveland Clinic ©2023

Causes

Bacteria in the mouth infect tissue surrounding the tooth, causing inflammation around the tooth leading to periodontal disease. When bacteria stay on the teeth long enough, they form a film called plaque, which eventually hardens to tartar, also called calculus. Tartar build-up can spread below the gum line, which makes the teeth harder to clean. Then, only a dental health professional can remove the tartar and stop the periodontal disease process.

Warning signs:

The following are warning signs of periodontal disease:

- Bad breath or bad taste that won't go away
- Red or swollen gums
- Tender or bleeding gums
- Painful chewing
- Loose teeth
- Sensitive teeth
- Gums that have pulled away from your teeth
- Any change in the way your teeth fit together when you bite
- Any change in the fit of partial dentures

Risk factors

Certain factors increase the risk for periodontal disease:

- Smoking
- Diabetes
- Poor oral hygiene
- Stress
- Heredity
- Crooked teeth
- Underlying immune-deficiencies e.g., AIDS
- Fillings that have become defective
- Taking medications that cause dry mouth
- Bridges that no longer fit properly
- Female hormonal changes, such as with pregnancy or the use of oral contraceptives

Prevention and Treatment

Gingivitis can be controlled and treated with good oral hygiene and regular professional cleaning. More severe forms of periodontal disease can also be treated successfully but may require more extensive treatment. Such treatment might include deep cleaning of the tooth root surfaces below the gums, medications prescribed to take by mouth or placed directly under the gums, and sometimes corrective surgery.

Why This Matters

You only get one body. Diseases don't happen overnight, and neither do solutions. Whether it's a cavity, gum disease, or another oral issue, it's all connected. Your oral health directly impacts your overall well-being.

It's not about perfection—it's about making informed choices every day. Listen to your body's signals, take small steps, and prioritize yourself.

Prevention: Small Habits, Big Impact

Prevention is alway better than the cure. It's easier to prevent oral health problems than to fix them later. Here's how:

1. **Brush and Floss Daily**
   Use a soft-bristled toothbrush and focus on your gum line. Don't forget to clean between teeth with floss or a water flosser.
2. **Maintain a Balanced Diet**
   Reduce sugar and acidic foods. Opt for vegetables, high-fiber foods, and water instead of sugary drinks.
3. **Breathe Through Your Nose**
   Mouth breathing dries out saliva, reducing its ability to neutralize harmful acids.
4. **Control pH Levels**
   Incorporate alkaline foods into your diet and use remineralizing toothpaste to protect enamel.
5. **Visit Your Dentist Regularly**
   Routine checkups can catch issues early before they become major problems.

If you can't afford dental care, you may be able to find help through the following sources:

The Health Resources and Services Administration supports a network of "safety net" clinics for people who qualify for reduced-cost care, and many have a dental clinic (toll free: 1-888-275-4772).

Starting Early: Pregnancy and Beyond

When planning for a family, most people focus on physical health, nutrition, and prenatal care but often overlook the role oral health plays in pregnancy outcomes and the long-term health of their child. Oral health during pregnancy affects more than just the mother's mouth; it can shape the development, health, and future of the baby.

Preparing for Pregnancy: Why Oral Health Matters

If you're planning to get pregnant, one of the best things you can do is schedule a dental checkup. Your oral health before pregnancy can influence your baby's development in ways most people don't realize.

How Oral Health Affects Your Baby

1. Preterm Birth and Low Birth Weight:
   Conditions like gum disease and untreated cavities can lead to inflammation and bacteria in the bloodstream, increasing the risk of premature delivery or low birth weight.
2. Nutritional Deficiency and Fetal Development:
   If the mother's oral health impacts her ability to chew, digest, or absorb nutrients, the baby may not get the essential vitamins and minerals needed for proper development.
3. The Oral Microbiome and Beyond:
   A healthy oral microbiome in the mother helps establish the child's microbiome. This microbiome affects everything from digestion to immune development.

Pregnancy Changes Everything—Including Your Mouth

Hormonal shifts during pregnancy can significantly affect oral health. For some women, pregnancy introduces no new issues, but for others, it exacerbates existing conditions or creates entirely new ones.

Common Oral Health Changes During Pregnancy

- Pregnancy Gingivitis:
  Hormonal changes can make gums more sensitive to plaque, leading to swelling, tenderness, and bleeding. If untreated, this can progress to more severe gum disease.
- Mouth Breathing and Snoring:
  Pregnancy can cause nasal congestion, leading to mouth breathing, which dries out saliva and increases the risk of cavities and gum disease.
- Clenching, Grinding, and Jaw Pain:
  Pregnancy-related stress or hormonal fluctuations can lead to increased clenching or grinding of teeth, putting strain on the jaw and teeth.
- Dry Mouth:
  Hormonal changes and increased hydration needs during pregnancy may cause dry mouth, reducing the natural cleansing effect of saliva.

Snoring, Sleep, and Pregnancy

Snoring and sleep-disordered breathing are surprisingly common during pregnancy, particularly in the third trimester. These issues can affect not only the mother's health but also the baby's development.

- How Snoring Impacts Pregnancy:
  - Reduced oxygen levels can increase risks of gestational hypertension, preeclampsia, and gestational diabetes.
  - Babies born to mothers with untreated sleep-disordered breathing are more likely to have lower birth weights.

What You Can Do:
If you snore or experience fatigue during pregnancy, talk to your healthcare provider. Simple interventions, such as a nasal spray or oral appliance, can improve airflow and sleep quality for both you and your baby.

Nutrition and Oral Health During Pregnancy

What you eat matters for your oral health and your baby's. Your baby's teeth begin forming between the third and sixth month of pregnancy, and certain nutrients are critical for their proper development.

Essential Nutrients for Oral Health:

- Calcium: For strong bones and teeth.
- Vitamin D: Helps your body absorb calcium effectively.
- Vitamin A: Supports enamel development.
- Vitamin C: Keeps gums healthy and supports connective tissues.

The Importance of Nasal Breathing During Pregnancy

Nasal breathing is often overlooked, but it plays a vital role in both oral and systemic health, especially during pregnancy.

Why Nasal Breathing Matters:

1. Improves Oxygenation: Proper oxygen flow supports both the mother's and baby's development.
2. Maintains Oral pH: Mouth breathing dries the mouth and disrupts its natural pH balance, increasing the risk of cavities and gum disease.
3. Supports Microbiome Health: The nasal microbiome contributes to the health of the oral microbiome and, by extension, the placental and fetal microbiomes.

Stories from Practice: How One Expectant Mother Changed Her Outcome

One of my patients, a first-time mom, came to me halfway through her pregnancy. She'd noticed her gums were bleeding and her jaw hurt every morning. She also admitted she had been snoring loudly and felt exhausted despite sleeping long hours.

When we looked closer, it turned out she was mouth breathing at night due to nasal congestion and grinding her teeth from stress. These two factors had contributed to early gum disease, which could put her at risk for a preterm birth.

With simple interventions like a nasal breathing strip, a custom night guard, and regular dental cleanings, she not only improved her oral health but also reported feeling more rested and energized. She delivered a full-term, healthy baby and said she'd never realized how connected her mouth was to her baby's health until she addressed these issues.

What to Watch for During Pregnancy

You should contact your dentist if you notice any of the following:

- Persistent gum bleeding or swelling
- Jaw pain or tooth sensitivity
- Snoring or frequent waking at night
- A sore in your mouth that doesn't heal within two weeks
- Toothaches or pain when chewing

Taking Charge of Your Oral Health

Your health is your baby's health. Here's how to take charge of your oral care during pregnancy:

1. Breathe Through Your Nose: If you experience nasal congestion, try a saline spray or talk to your provider about other safe solutions.
2. Brush and Floss Daily: Use a soft-bristled toothbrush and fluoride toothpaste to keep gums healthy.
3. Stay Hydrated: Drink plenty of water to promote saliva production and keep bacteria at bay.
4. Visit Your Dentist Regularly: Make sure your dentist knows you're pregnant and keep up with cleanings and exams.
5. Monitor Your Diet: Choose foods that support oral and overall health, such as leafy greens, dairy products, and lean proteins.

A Healthy Mouth, A Healthy Baby

Your mouth is the foundation for your overall health, and during pregnancy, it's also the starting point for your baby's development. By taking care of your oral health before, during, and after pregnancy, you're giving your child the best possible start to a healthy life.

Mouth breathing during pregnancy is not just an inconvenience it can have profound effects on both the mother's health and the baby's growth and development.

How Mouth Breathing Affects Pregnancy:

Mouth breathing disrupts the natural balance in the body, leading to a cascade of effects:

1. Reduced Oxygen Levels:
   Oxygen is essential for the mother's body to function optimally during pregnancy. Chronic mouth breathing reduces oxygen intake, which can lead to maternal fatigue, headaches, and even complications like gestational hypertension or preeclampsia.
2. Disrupted Oral Microbiome:
   Mouth breathing dries out saliva, disrupting the oral microbiome. This can lead to an increased risk of cavities, gum disease, and systemic inflammation, all of which can impact the pregnancy.
3. Increased Risk of Snoring and Sleep Apnea:
   Mouth breathing is often associated with snoring and obstructive sleep apnea (OSA). OSA in pregnant women has been linked to higher rates of preterm labor, gestational diabetes, and cesarean delivery.

The Baby's Health: Low Birth Weight and Development

Mouth breathing during pregnancy has been shown to directly affect fetal growth and development. Here's how:

1. Low Birth Weight:
   Studies have found that babies born to mothers with untreated snoring, sleep-disordered breathing, or chronic mouth breathing are more likely to have low birth weight. Low birth weight is associated with an increased risk of developmental delays, compromised immune systems, and long-term health issues like diabetes and cardiovascular disease.
2. Oxygen Deprivation:
   When the mother doesn't receive adequate oxygen due to mouth breathing, the baby's oxygen supply is also compromised. This can affect organ development, brain growth, and overall fetal health.

3. Altered Growth Patterns:

Chronic mouth breathing in mothers can influence the baby's craniofacial growth. A baby exposed to poor oxygenation may have altered bone and muscle development, potentially predisposing them to airway and orthodontic issues later in life.

4. Impact on the Placental Microbiome:

The mother's oral and nasal microbiomes influence the placental microbiome. Mouth breathing disrupts the balance of bacteria, which can lead to inflammation and affect the nutrient supply to the baby.

Preventing the Effects of Mouth Breathing During Pregnancy

The good news is that there are simple steps mothers can take to minimize the impact of mouth breathing on their health and their baby's development:

1. Address the Cause of Mouth Breathing
- Nasal Congestion Relief:
  - Use a saline spray or humidifier to reduce nasal inflammation.
  - Nasal strips can also improve airflow and encourage nasal breathing.
- Allergy Management:
  If allergies are contributing to mouth breathing, consult your healthcare provider for safe remedies during pregnancy.

2. Seek Help for Sleep Issues
- Sleep Studies:
  If you snore or feel excessively tired, talk to your healthcare provider about a sleep study to rule out obstructive sleep apnea.
- Oral Appliances:
  Temporary oral appliances can support the airway and encourage nasal breathing during pregnancy.

3. Practice Good Oral Hygiene
- Use a fluoride toothpaste and rinse to minimize the effects of dry mouth caused by mouth breathing.
- Stay hydrated to support saliva production and maintain a healthy oral pH balance.

4. Prioritize Nasal Breathing

- Breathing Exercises:
  Techniques like Buteyko breathing can train the body to rely more on nasal breathing.
- Myofunctional Therapy:
  Working with a myofunctional therapist can address tongue posture and retrain the muscles involved in breathing.

A Case for Awareness

One patient shared her experience of waking up daily with a dry mouth, swollen gums, and significant fatigue. She dismissed these as typical pregnancy symptoms until her third trimester, when her baby was diagnosed as being small for gestational age. Further investigation revealed that her mouth breathing was contributing to sleep apnea and reducing her oxygen levels at night.

With simple interventions like nasal strips and daily breathing exercises, her oxygen levels improved, and she delivered a healthy baby at 38 weeks. She now advocates for better awareness of mouth breathing and its impact during pregnancy.

Why Early Action Matters

Awareness of mouth breathing and its impact on pregnancy outcomes is still emerging. However, the evidence is clear: addressing this issue early can lead to better outcomes for both Mother and baby. A focus on nasal breathing, oral hygiene, and overall airway health can:

- Reduce the risk of low birth weight.
- Support proper fetal development.
- Improve maternal energy and reduce pregnancy complications.

A healthy pregnancy begins with a healthy airway. By addressing mouth breathing and its related issues, you're taking a significant step toward giving your baby the best start in life.

Remember, you have the power to shape your and your baby's future starting with the care you give your mouth. Through my proprietary course, you'll be guided step-by-step from before birth and beyond using The S.M.I.L.E. System: Support, Milestones, Inform, Learn, Empower. Together, we'll build a foundation for lifelong health, one habit at a time.

CHAPTER 9

Personalized Health:
Testing, Prevention and Daily Practices

Beyond One-Size-Fits-All: A Critique of Current Healthcare Approaches.

The current healthcare approach, particularly in Western medicine, is often criticized for being highly fragmented, reactive, and focused primarily on symptom management rather than prevention or holistic well-being.

Here are some key critiques of the current healthcare system:

1. Fragmented Care

While healthcare has advanced treatment in specific areas, it has also created a fragmented system where healthcare providers treat the body in isolated parts rather than as an interconnected whole. Specialists often focus on their area of expertise whether it's the heart, lungs, or teeth without fully understanding or addressing how these systems influence each other.

- Example: A dentist might treat cavities or gum disease without considering the patient's breathing habits, airway, nutrition, hydration, or sleep which could be contributing factors. Similarly, a cardiologist might prescribe medication for high blood pressure without considering how the patient's sleep or stress levels are impacting their cortisol levels and overall health.

This fragmentation often results in missed opportunities for early intervention, prevention and diagnosis because doctors aren't viewing the body as a connected system.

2. Reactive Rather Than Proactive

The current healthcare system tends to focus on treating diseases and symptoms after they arise, rather than preventing them in the first place. Most healthcare interventions occur when patients are already symptomatic, which often means that chronic diseases like diabetes, heart disease, or even oral health problems are caught after considerable damage has been done.

- Example: Instead of educating patients on preventive lifestyle changes such as diet, exercise, breathing, and stress management, many doctors are more likely to prescribe medications to manage symptoms of chronic diseases. This approach doesn't address the root causes and can lead to patients becoming reliant on medication rather than making lasting health improvements.

Prevention and education, especially in areas like nutrition, oral health, sleep, and mental well-being, are often overlooked or underemphasized.

3. Lack of Integration Between Mind, Body, Mouth and Oral Health

Current healthcare models often fail to acknowledge the critical connection between mental health, physical health, and oral health. While these aspects of health are deeply intertwined, they are frequently treated as separate entities.

- Mental and Physical Health: Many medical treatments focus solely on physical symptoms without addressing the psychological or emotional factors that contribute to illness. For instance, stress and anxiety can exacerbate conditions like high blood pressure or sleep disorders, but addressing these mental health issues isn't always a primary concern in treatment plans.
- Oral Health as an Afterthought: Oral health is often relegated to a secondary concern, despite its well-documented connection to systemic health issues such as cardiovascular disease, diabetes, and even cognitive decline. The mouth is the gateway to the body, yet it's rarely included in broader healthcare conversations.

4. One-Size-Fits-All Approach

Many healthcare treatments take a one-size-fits-all approach, prescribing standardized protocols that don't account for individual differences in genetics, lifestyle, sensitivities or personal health histories. This is particularly concerning when treating chronic illnesses, which can have varied causes and responses to treatment across different individuals.

- Example: Two people with the same diagnosis of hypertension might be treated with the same medication, even though their underlying causes (stress, diet, genetics, sleep, etc.) may be entirely different. This approach fails to personalize treatment and overlooks the need for a more tailored approach to each individual's health.

The healthcare system tends to focus on managing symptoms rather than exploring the root causes that could differ significantly from one patient to another.

5. Over Reliance on Medication

While medication is essential for treating certain conditions, there is an overreliance on pharmaceuticals in modern healthcare. Instead of promoting lifestyle changes, doctors often prescribe medication as the first line of defense against chronic conditions like hypertension, anxiety, depression, or even oral health issues.

- Example: For patients with high blood pressure or diabetes, medications like beta-blockers or insulin might be prescribed, but these don't address the underlying issues of diet, stress, or sleep that could be causing the problem. This often leads to lifelong dependency on medication without addressing the root causes and possible side effects of medications.

While medications can save lives, this approach neglects the potential for lifestyle and holistic interventions to mitigate or even reverse certain conditions.

6. Inaccessible and Inequitable Healthcare

Another significant critique is the inaccessibility of healthcare, especially in the United States. Millions of people do not have adequate healthcare coverage, which leaves them unable to access preventive care, routine check-ups, or early treatment. This not only exacerbates health conditions but also disproportionately impacts low-income and marginalized communities. Or they are paying so much just to have insurance they do not use it due to co-pays on top of expenses.

- Example: Preventive services such as dental check-ups, nutritional counseling, or mental health support may be out of reach for individuals without sufficient health insurance. This leads to untreated conditions escalating into more severe health crises, which then require more intensive and expensive care.

7. Lack of Focus on Patient Education

The current healthcare system often fails to empower patients with the knowledge and tools to manage their own health. Doctors may prescribe treatments or recommend lifestyle changes, but the time and resources to truly educate patients on why these changes matter and how to implement them are often lacking.

- Example: A doctor might tell a patient to "reduce stress," but without offering specific tools or techniques (like breathing exercises, mindfulness, or physical activity), patients may not know how to make meaningful changes. This lack of education can lead to patients feeling disempowered and dependent on the healthcare system for long-term health management.

8. Ignoring Basic Human Needs

Healthcare systems frequently ignore the most basic, yet fundamental, aspects of human health: proper hydration, nutrition, sleep, and breathing. These foundational elements are often assumed to be the patient's responsibility without offering the necessary support or resources to address them in a meaningful way.

- Example: Conditions such as sleep apnea, dehydration, poor diet, and chronic stress are seldom addressed in routine medical visits, even though they are major contributors to chronic disease. Yet, small improvements in these areas can lead to profound health outcomes.

9. High Cost and Burnout in Healthcare Professionals

The healthcare system's emphasis on treating symptoms through diagnostics, surgeries, and medications has not only become costly but also leads to physician burnout. Doctors are pressured to see more patients in less time, limiting their ability to build meaningful relationships or spend time exploring preventive measures with their patients.

- Example: Overworked healthcare providers may not have the time to offer holistic advice or follow up on lifestyle interventions, relying instead on quick fixes like medication or referrals to specialists. This transactional model of care further exacerbates the disconnect between patient and provider.

Moving forward:

To address these the future of healthcare needs to shift toward a more integrative, holistic, and preventive model that recognizes the connection between the mind, mouth, and body. This approach would:

- Prioritize prevention and education, helping patients understand how their daily choices like nutrition, hydration, sleep, and stress management affect their overall health.
- Collaboration among healthcare providers, ensuring that professionals from various disciplines work together to treat the whole person, not just isolated symptoms.
- Encourage personalized care, taking into account each individual's unique health history, lifestyle, and needs.
- Address the root causes of chronic disease rather than simply managing symptoms with medication.

By acknowledging the critical connections between various aspects of health and focusing on holistic, patient-centered care, the healthcare system can begin to treat the whole person and promote long-term wellness, rather than simply reacting to disease.

Importance of personalized health assessments.

The importance of personalized health assessments cannot be overstated. Personalized health assessments consider the unique physical, mental, and lifestyle factors that contribute to an individual's health, offering a more accurate and effective approach to prevention, diagnosis, and treatment. This tailored approach is crucial for achieving optimal health outcomes and empowering individuals to take charge of their own well-being.

Here's why personalized health assessments are so essential in today's healthcare landscape:

1. Recognizing Individual Differences

Every person is unique, with different genetic backgrounds, lifestyles, environmental exposures, and health histories. These variations mean that even people with the same diagnosis or health concerns may require different treatment approaches. Personalized health assessments take into account these differences, offering tailored insights that go beyond generic health advice.

2. Preventive Health Through Early Detection

Personalized health assessments often involve in-depth evaluations of risk factors, genetics, and lifestyle habits, allowing for the early detection of potential health issues before they manifest as symptoms. This proactive approach helps individuals take preventive measures to maintain their health and avoid more serious complications down the road.

- Example: A personalized health assessment might reveal that an individual is at higher risk for diabetes based on family history, diet, and blood sugar levels. This early identification allows for preventive interventions such as dietary changes, exercise, and weight management, potentially delaying or even preventing the onset of the disease.

3. Targeted Health Interventions

When health assessments are personalized, they provide a roadmap for targeted interventions. Rather than relying on generalized treatment protocols, healthcare providers can design specific plans that align with an individual's health needs, maximizing the chances of success.

- Example: If a personalized health assessment reveals that a patient's stress is significantly affecting their sleep and overall health, the healthcare provider can recommend targeted interventions like breathing exercises, mindfulness practices, and sleep hygiene strategies. This approach directly addresses the patient's root problems rather than just treating symptoms with medication.

4. Addressing Mental, Emotional, and Environmental Factors

Health is not just about the physical body; it's also shaped by mental, emotional, and environmental factors. Personalized health assessments take these dimensions into account, offering a more holistic view of an individual's well-being. By addressing stress, mental health, sleep patterns, and environmental influences, these assessments provide a fuller picture of what's contributing to or hindering optimal health.

- Example: A personalized health assessment might reveal that a person's anxiety or chronic stress is affecting their digestion, immune system, or sleep quality. By recognizing this link, healthcare providers can recommend interventions like counseling, stress management, or lifestyle adjustments that address the root cause rather than just treating the symptoms.

5. Empowering Individuals to Take Ownership of Their Health

Personalized health assessments empower individuals by providing them with a clear understanding of their unique health status and risks. This knowledge encourages people to take ownership of their health, make informed decisions, and take proactive steps toward better well-being.

- Example: When patients are given detailed insights about their health, they are more likely to follow through with lifestyle changes or treatments. A personalized assessment might highlight how a person's hydration habits, sleep patterns, or nutrition are affecting their overall health, motivating them to make positive adjustments with confidence.

- Example: If a personalized assessment reveals that a patient's chronic headaches are linked to poor posture, stress, and inadequate hydration, the treatment plan can address each of these factors in a coordinated manner, offering a more comprehensive solution than treating the headache alone.

Action Steps:

When it comes to taking charge of your health or promoting personalized health assessments, here are a few other key things you need to know:

1. The Importance of Data and Technology

- Wearable Health Tech: Devices like fitness trackers, smartwatches, and apps that monitor your health metrics (sleep, heart rate, stress levels, etc.) are becoming more common and can provide valuable data for personalized health assessments.
- Genetic Testing: Services like 23andMe or DNAfit offer genetic insights that can guide personalized health plans, particularly in areas like nutrition, exercise, and disease prevention.
- Telemedicine: As telehealth grows, remote consultations combined with data from wearable devices are making personalized assessments more accessible. Make sure you're aware of the technologies available that can help track, analyze, and optimize your health.

2. Environmental and Lifestyle Factors

- Work Environment: Consider how your workplace setup or habits may affect your overall health. Long hours sitting, high stress, poor air quality, and limited access to nutritious food can all play roles in your health.
- Home Environment: Pay attention to things like sleep hygiene, exposure to pollutants or allergens, and overall comfort at home, as these factors directly impact your well-being.
- Exercise and Movement: Regular movement beyond structured exercise is crucial. Simple activities like walking, stretching, or incorporating "micro-movements" throughout the day can greatly affect your overall health.

3. The Role of Stress and Mental Health

- Chronic Stress: Long-term stress has profound effects on your body, leading to conditions like hypertension, heart disease, digestive problems, and even mental health disorders. Mindfulness practices, breathing exercises, and relaxation techniques are essential in personalized health plans.
- Emotional Wellness: Your mental and emotional well-being directly impacts your physical health. Issues like anxiety, depression, and unresolved trauma can contribute to chronic health conditions.

4. Hydration and pH Balance

- Water Intake: Dehydration affects everything from your energy levels to digestion and cognitive function. Ensuring you get enough water each day is essential for maintaining a healthy body.
- pH Balance: The acidity or alkalinity of your body plays a role in inflammation, digestion, and disease prevention. Maintaining a balanced pH level through proper hydration, diet (with emphasis on alkaline foods), and reducing stress can prevent diseases and optimize health.

5. Gut Health

- Microbiome Importance: The health of your gut directly impacts your immune system, digestion, and even mental health. Personalized health assessments should take into account factors like diet, stress, and medications that affect your gut microbiome.
- Probiotics and Prebiotics: Including gut-friendly foods, such as fermented products (probiotics) and fiber-rich foods (prebiotics), can improve digestion and overall health.

6. Sleep Quality and Quantity

- Sleep Hygiene: The importance of sleep for overall health cannot be overstated. Many people focus on diet and exercise but overlook the critical role of high-quality sleep. Ensuring a consistent sleep schedule, reducing screen time before bed, and creating a relaxing sleep environment are foundational steps.
- Sleep Apnea and Disorders: Be aware of sleep conditions like sleep apnea, which can severely impact health if left untreated. Personalized health assessments should include evaluations of sleep patterns and quality to help address sleep-related issues.

7. Preventive Healthcare Screenings

- Regular Check-ups: Even when focusing on holistic health, regular check-ups with healthcare professionals for early detection of potential issues are essential. Blood tests, hormone panels, and physical exams provide valuable information about your overall health.

- Cancer Screenings: Be proactive with preventive screenings for cancers like breast, prostate, colon, and skin, especially if there's a family history. There are blood and other tests that can detect cancer early.

8. Oral Health's Role in Overall Well-being

- Oral-Systemic Connection: Your mouth is a window into your overall health. Gum disease and other oral health issues have been linked to heart disease, diabetes, and even Alzheimer's. Make sure oral health is included in personalized assessments to prevent systemic health problems.
- Nasal Breathing and Sleep: Breathing through your nose instead of your mouth while sleeping can improve sleep quality and reduce the risk of sleep apnea, which has further implications for heart health and cognitive function.

9. Sustainable Habits Over Quick Fixes

- Consistency Over Perfection: Long-term health is about making sustainable, consistent changes rather than drastic, short-term fixes. Whether it's diet, exercise, or stress management, success comes from integrating small, manageable changes over time.
- Adaptable Plans: Life circumstances change, and so should your health plan. Personalized health assessments should be adaptable to account for new stressors, changes in lifestyle, or different health needs as you age.

10. Holistic Approach to Chronic Disease Management

- Multifactorial Treatment Plans: Chronic diseases like diabetes, hypertension, and arthritis are often treated with medications, but a personalized health plan would take a more comprehensive approach. By considering breathing, diet, movement, stress management, sleep, and oral health, you can often reduce symptoms or slow disease progression naturally.

Testing, Not Guessing:

Benefits of Individualized Testing for Targeted Treatment

Individualized testing, often referred to as personalized or precision medicine, involves using specific diagnostic tests tailored to a person's unique genetic, biological, and lifestyle factors. This approach enables healthcare providers to design highly targeted treatment plans that address the root causes of a patient's condition rather than relying on one-size-fits-all solutions. Below are some of the key benefits of individualized testing for targeted treatment:

1. Accurate Diagnosis and Treatment
2. Personalized Treatment Plans
3. Reduced Side Effects
4. Improved Outcomes
5. Prevention of Disease Progression
6. Cost-Effective Care
7. Reduction in Trial-and-Error Prescribing
8. Preventive and Proactive Health Management
9. Increased Patient Engagement and Satisfaction
10. Holistic Understanding of Health

Individualized testing offers a comprehensive view of the patient's health, incorporating genetic, biochemical, environmental, and lifestyle factors into the diagnosis and treatment plan. This holistic approach goes beyond just treating the symptoms and helps to address the root causes of health problems.

Individualized testing is a game-changer in modern healthcare, offering a more precise, effective, and patient-centered approach to diagnosis and treatment. By taking into account a person's unique genetic, biological, and lifestyle factors, targeted treatments can deliver better health outcomes, fewer side effects, and a more proactive approach to preventing disease. As healthcare moves toward a more personalized model, individualized testing will continue to play a crucial role in optimizing patient care.

The future of healthcare should shift toward an integrative, holistic model that acknowledges the connections between mind, mouth, and body. This approach would prioritize prevention, collaboration among healthcare providers, and personalized care to address root causes rather than merely managing symptoms. By focusing on holistic, patient-centered care, the healthcare system can promote long-term wellness and prevent chronic disease rather than simply reacting to it.

Practical Steps for Daily Health:

Creating a daily routine that integrates holistic health practices can help support overall wellness by addressing the mind, body, and oral health connection. Here's a well-rounded daily routine to improve your health, focusing on breathing, nutrition, hydration, sleep, and self-care:

Morning Routine (Start Your Day Right)

1. Mindful Breathing (5-10 minutes)
   - Begin your day with a few minutes of deep, mindful breathing to reduce stress and activate your parasympathetic nervous system.
   - Technique: Try the 4-7-8 breathing method (inhale for 4 seconds, hold for 7 seconds, exhale for 8 seconds). This promotes relaxation and better focus for the day ahead.
2. Nasal Hygiene
   - Clear your nasal passages with a saline rinse or neti pot to support optimal breathing throughout the day. Proper nasal breathing helps maintain oxygen balance and improves focus and energy levels.
3. Hydrate (Start with Water)
   - Drink a full glass of water first thing in the morning. Add a slice of lemon for an alkalizing boost to help balance your body's pH levels and kickstart hydration.
4. Oral Health Care (2-3 minutes)
   - Brush your teeth and floss to support your oral health. Consider using a tongue scraper to remove bacteria and improve overall mouth hygiene.
   - Tip: Nasal breathing helps with oral health by reducing the risk of dry mouth and improving sleep quality.
5. Movement (15-20 minutes)

- Engage in light movement to wake up your body, whether it's stretching, yoga, or a walk outside. Physical activity boosts circulation, reduces stiffness, and enhances mental clarity.
6. Nourishing Breakfast
   - Focus on a balanced meal that includes whole foods rich in fiber, protein, and healthy fats. Incorporate greens and lean proteins to fuel your body and promote stable energy levels throughout the day.

Mid-Morning (Boost Focus and Energy)

1. Hydrate Throughout the Morning
   - Drink water consistently throughout the morning. Aim for 1-2 cups before lunch to keep your body hydrated.
2. Nasal Breathing Check
   - Perform nasal breathing throughout the day to ensure deep, controlled breaths. Avoid mouth breathing, which can lead to fatigue and lower oxygen intake.
3. Take Movement Breaks
   - Every hour, take a few minutes to stand, stretch, and move. Incorporating short movement breaks throughout the day improves circulation and mental focus.

Lunchtime Routine (Re-energize)

1. Mindful Eating
   - Eat a balanced meal with plenty of vegetables, lean protein, and whole grains. Avoid processed foods or heavy meals that can sap energy.
   - Practice mindful eating by chewing slowly and focusing on the textures and flavors of your food to support digestion and prevent overeating.
2. Hydration Boost
   - Drink water or herbal tea during and after lunch to stay hydrated.
3. Midday Breathing Break (5 minutes)

- Take a quick break after lunch to do a few rounds of deep breathing. This helps manage stress and refocuses your mind for the afternoon ahead.

Afternoon Routine (Sustain Energy)

1. Stay Hydrated
   - Keep drinking water throughout the afternoon, aiming for another 2-3 cups. Hydration supports mental clarity and prevents afternoon slumps.
2. Short Physical Activity (10-15 minutes)
   - Incorporate a short walk or stretching break to re-energize and prevent stiffness from sitting too long.
3. Power Snack
   - If needed, have a small, nutritious snack in the afternoon, such as nuts, fruit, or yogurt. This will help sustain your energy until dinner without a sugar crash.

Evening Routine (Wind Down)

1. Unplug from Screens
   - Avoid screen time (TV, phone, computer) at least an hour before bed to prevent disruptions in your sleep cycle from blue light exposure.
2. Calming Activity
   - Engage in a relaxing activity like reading, journaling, or meditation. This helps calm your mind and prepares you for restful sleep.
3. Oral Hygiene (2-3 minutes)
   - Before bed, brush and floss your teeth to maintain good oral health. Consider using an alcohol-free mouthwash to keep your gums and mouth clean overnight.
4. Hydration Check
   - Drink a small glass of water before bed but avoid large amounts that could disrupt your sleep.
5. Gratitude Practice or Reflection (5 minutes)

- Spend a few minutes reflecting on the positive moments of your day. Writing down three things you're grateful for or reviewing your day mindfully can help reduce stress and set a positive tone before sleep.
6. Nasal Breathing for Sleep (5 minutes)
   - Before bed, practice deep nasal breathing to activate the relaxation response and prepare for sleep. This helps to reduce cortisol levels and promotes deeper, restorative sleep.

Bedtime (Sleep Hygiene and Recovery)

1. Sleep Environment
   - Ensure your bedroom is cool, dark, and quiet to optimize sleep. Remove electronic devices from the room to avoid distractions and blue light.
2. Set a Consistent Sleep Schedule
   - Aim for 7-9 hours of sleep each night. Going to bed and waking up at the same time daily helps regulate your internal clock and improves sleep quality.

Additional Weekly Practices

1. Meal Planning and Preparation

Take some time each week to plan and prepare balanced, nutritious meals that support your overall health goals. Incorporating fresh, whole foods and reducing processed items can make a big difference in your energy and mood throughout the week.

2. Weekly Review and Adjustment

Reflect on your habits at the end of the week and adjust accordingly. Are you staying consistent with hydration, movement, and stress management? Identify areas that need improvement and set small, manageable goals for the following week.

This daily routine focuses on integrating key habits breathing, hydration, movement, nutrition, sleep, and oral health into your life. By following these small but impactful practices, you can optimize your physical, mental, and overall well-being.

Prevention Over Cure:

The importance of proactive health measures.

> Proactive health measures are essential for preventing disease and promoting long-term well-being. By taking steps such as maintaining a balanced diet, staying physically active, practicing good oral hygiene, managing stress, and getting regular check-ups, individuals can address potential health issues before they become serious. These measures empower people to take control of their health, reduce the risk of chronic diseases, and improve their overall quality of life. Proactive care not only leads to better outcomes but also reduces the need for costly medical interventions down the line.

Continually Educate Yourself

> Stay Informed: Keep learning about new developments in health, wellness, and nutrition. Read books, attend workshops, and stay engaged with the latest health research.

> Listen to Your Body: Pay attention to how your body responds to different foods, activities, or stressors, and adjust your routine as needed. Health is dynamic, so regularly evaluate what works.

Build Sustainable, Long-Term Habits

> Small, Consistent Changes: Focus on making small but consistent changes over time rather than seeking quick fixes or short-term trends. Long-term health is achieved through daily habits that become part of your lifestyle.

> Flexibility and Adaptation: Be adaptable as your needs change over time. What works for you in your 20s may differ in your 40s, 50's or 60's so stay flexible and evolve your habits as needed to fit your current circumstances.

CHAPTER 10

Conclusion

Your Health, Your Responsibility: Empowerment and Ownership

Taking ownership of your health is not just a necessity but an empowering step toward living a more vibrant and fulfilling life. When you take charge of your well-being, you gain control over the choices that influence your body, mind, and long-term health. It's about recognizing every decision from what you eat to how you manage stress and what you feel. Health is not a passive experience, and by taking responsibility, you can prevent disease, enhance your quality of life, and build resilience against the inevitable challenges that life presents. Live the life you want.

Recap: The Importance of Taking Ownership of Health

Owning your health means embracing a proactive approach. It's about preventing disease before it starts, rather than waiting for symptoms to emerge. Through simple, daily actions like nourishing your body with balanced nutrition, staying hydrated, managing stress, moving regularly, and prioritizing sleep, you can drastically improve your overall wellness. Your health is a reflection of the habits you cultivate small steps lead to big changes over time. When you take ownership of your health, you become an active participant in your well-being, empowered to make choices that align with the life you want to live.

Encouragement and Final Thoughts

Remember, no one knows your body better than you do. You have the power to make the necessary changes and choices that will keep you healthy, strong, and thriving. It's never too late to begin, whether you're just starting or looking to reinforce habits you've already established. Start where you are now! True wellness is a journey, not a destination, and each step you take toward better health is a victory worth celebrating.

You are not alone on this journey there are countless resources, professionals, and tools available to guide and support you. Take pride in the fact that every effort you make is an investment in your future self. It's not about perfection; it's about progress, and every positive change is a step toward a healthier, more fulfilling life.

The Health Benefits of Smiling

Smiles last a lifetime, the more you have the happier your life will be. It seems simple, life gets hard sometimes. Going back to the basics O.W.N.E.R is always a great place not only to start but to go back to if your life feels overwhelming. How you feel, your emotions and your thoughts are what dictate the kind of life you will live.

We are taught not to be selfish, but selfish is exactly what we need to be. Selfish with our energy, with who we give our time to and with establishing healthy boundaries.

We would do much better in life if we were taught at a younger age to figure out what that means to us. Most of us have no idea until later in life what even makes us happy. I had no idea all of the options available. Smiling is your superpower. A smile spurs a powerful chemical reaction in the brain that can make you feel happier. Your body releases three hormones that make you feel good when you smile. They include dopamine, endorphins and serotonin.

"Life is like a mirror, smile at it and it smiles back at you"

They say it takes more muscles to frown than to smile, and although there's no hard evidence to support that, we do know that smiling comes with some real-life benefits.

It's not always the easiest thing to do, especially after a loss or a long and stressful day. But if you can take it upon yourself to crack a smile, you'll actually feel better.

One study even suggests that smiling can help us recover faster from stress and reduce our heart rate. In fact, it might even be worth your while to fake a smile and see how you feel.

Creating a Ripple Effect or a Butterfly Effect as I call it

The benefits of smiling aren't just limited to yourself it can also affect those around you. When we smile, we're also rewarded when we see someone else smile. Try it, if they do not smile back they are deep in thought. A different part of the brain has to engage for them not to crack a smile.

The reward center of our brain is activated with a smile and it makes us feel a little better. One Swedish study suggests that we can't help but react with a smile of our own when we see someone smiling.

Final Call to Action

Today is the perfect day to take control of your health. Start small, build momentum, and watch how these changes transform your life. Whether it's prioritizing your sleep, practicing mindful breathing, or making healthier food choices, every action counts. Take ownership of your health, empower yourself with knowledge, and make choices that align with the life you envision. Your health is your responsibility, and with it comes the power to live your best life. Be proactive rather than reactive.

You are in control so take that first step, today. There is no time like the present. They call it the present because it is a gift.

You are the only OWNER of your health and the impact of small, consistent changes over time is priceless.

CHAPTER 11

Case Studies: Real Lives Transformed

The Power of Proper Diagnosis

Sarah's Story: More Than Just ADHD

When Sarah's mother brought her 8-year-old daughter to my office, they had already spent two years trying different ADHD medications. Sarah was struggling in school despite being bright, and her behavior was affecting the whole family. What traditional evaluations missed was that Sarah was a chronic mouth breather with an undiagnosed tongue tie.

After proper sleep testing revealed sleep-disordered breathing:

- Her mouth breathing was addressed
- Tongue tie was treated
- Myofunctional therapy was implemented
- Sleep quality improved dramatically

Within six months:

- School performance improved
- Behavior stabilized
- ADHD medication was no longer needed
- Family life transformed

When Results Don't Tell the Whole Story

Looking Beyond Numbers

Why Standard Tests Can Miss Important Issues:

1. One-night studies don't show the full picture
2. Unfamiliar environments affect sleep patterns
3. Standard metrics don't capture all breathing issues
4. Children often present differently than adults

Red Flags to Watch For Despite "Normal" Results:

- Continued daytime fatigue
- Persistent mouth breathing
- Dental issues developing
- Behavioral concerns
- Morning symptoms

Additional Assessments to Consider:

1. Airway evaluation
2. Dental arch examination
3. Tongue function assessment
4. Breathing pattern analysis

Creating Your Support Team:

- Sleep specialist
- Dental professional
- Myofunctional therapist
- Primary care physician
- Other specialists as needed

What Was Missed: Chronic mouth breathing, frequent micro-arousals, and a tongue-tie.

What Was Given: Nasal hygiene, tongue-tie release, and myofunctional therapy.

Outcome: Sarah's focus improved, her behavior stabilized, and her ADHD medication was discontinued within six months.

Success Stories: The Many Faces of Sleep Issues

The "Problem Child" Who Wasn't: Tommy's Story

When Tommy's parents came to me, they were at their wit's end. Their 6-year-old had been kicked out of two schools, was on multiple behavioral medications, and the family was falling apart. His mother's intuition told her something wasn't right, but no one would listen.

Initial assessments showed:

- Dark circles under eyes
- Mouth breathing
- Forward head posture
- Difficulty focusing
- Bedwetting
- Night terrors

Standard sleep testing showed only mild issues, but further investigation revealed:

- Significant tongue tie
- Narrow dental arches
- Compromised airway
- Chronic mouth breathing

After comprehensive treatment:

- Behavior improved dramatically
- School performance transformed
- Bedwetting resolved
- Family life restored
- Medications reduced then eliminated

The Quiet Sufferer: Emma's Story

Not all children with sleep problems act out. Some, like Emma, suffer in silence, and these cases are often the most overlooked. Emma was a 9-year-old girl who did everything "right." She got good grades, never caused trouble in class, and was always helpful at home. She was the kind of student teachers dream of having in their classroom.

The Hidden Signs

What brought Emma to my office wasn't behavioral issues—it was a routine dental check-up where I noticed:

- Severe teeth grinding

- Worn down enamel
- A high, narrow palate
- Slightly dark circles under her eyes
- Perfect, quiet behavior (almost too perfect)

During my examination, Emma's mother mentioned casually, "She's always been such a good sleeper. Goes to bed without complaint and we never hear a peep from her all night."

Digging Deeper

When I started asking more questions, a different picture emerged:

- Emma needed 12 hours of sleep to feel rested
- She was impossible to wake in the morning
- She fell asleep instantly at bedtime (a red flag—normal sleepers take 15-20 minutes)
- She never moved during sleep (another red flag—healthy sleepers move periodically)
- She had frequent headaches but never complained
- Her sheets were soaked with sweat every morning
- She was in the 5th percentile for weight despite eating well

The Assessment

Further evaluation revealed:

- Severe upper airway resistance
- Chronic mouth breathing during sleep
- Microarousals happening hundreds of times per night
- Oxygen saturation drops that weren't severe enough to register as concerning on standard tests
- A tongue tie that had been missed by multiple healthcare providers

Why It Was Missed

Emma's case had been overlooked because:

1. She performed well academically

2. She didn't snore loudly
3. She didn't display behavioral issues
4. She never complained
5. She appeared to sleep through the night
6. Standard pediatric check-ups didn't catch the subtle signs

The Treatment Journey

Working with a team of professionals, we:

1. Addressed the tongue tie
2. Implemented myofunctional therapy
3. Worked on proper tongue positioning
4. Established nasal breathing patterns
5. Started palatal expansion
6. Created healthy sleep hygiene practices

The Transformation

Within six months:

- Emma's energy levels soared
- Her headaches disappeared
- She started growing rapidly
- Her dark circles faded
- Morning wake-ups became easier
- Her quiet personality remained, but with newfound vitality
- Her mother reported, "It's like she was living in black and white before, and now she's in color."

The Lessons

Emma's case taught us several crucial points:

1. Good behavior doesn't always mean good sleep
2. Quiet sufferers often go undiagnosed the longest
3. "Perfect" children sometimes need the most help
4. Standard sleep studies don't catch everything
5. Multiple subtle signs can add up to a significant problem

What Was Missed: Mouth breathing, upper airway resistance, and fragmented sleep.

What Was Given: Nasal breathing training and palatal expansion.

Outcome: Emma's energy and mood improved, and her headaches disappeared.

Warning Signs for Quiet Sufferers:

- Excessive sleep needs
- Morning headaches
- Night sweats
- Instant sleep onset
- Lack of movement during sleep
- Consistent dark circles
- Unexplained growth delays
- "Perfect" behavior
- Daytime fatigue masked as calmness
- Teeth grinding

This case revolutionized how I screen all children, not just those with obvious symptoms. It's why I now tell parents: Don't wait for problems to become severe or obvious. The quiet sufferers remind us that sometimes the children who appear to be doing the best on the surface are struggling the most underneath.

The Gifted Student: Michael's Story

Michael was already at the top of his class when he came to my office. A 15-year-old sophomore taking advanced placement classes, president of the debate team, and aspiring medical student. His parents brought him in for a routine dental check-up, not because they thought anything was wrong—after all, he was excelling in every way.

The Unexpected Discovery

During the examination, I noticed:

- Slight teeth wear patterns
- A narrow smile

- Forward head posture
- Pen chewing habits
- Fidgeting with his hands
- Dark circles under his eyes (masked by his glasses)

The "Normal" Day

Michael's typical schedule:

- Up at 5:30 AM for early morning study
- School from 7:30 AM - 3:00 PM
- Extracurricular activities until 6:00 PM
- Homework until midnight
- "Running on caffeine and determination"

His mother proudly shared, "He's always been driven. Even as a toddler, he never napped—just kept going and going."

Diving Deeper

Despite his academic success, certain patterns emerged:

- Needed multiple alarms to wake up
- Consumed 4-5 energy drinks daily
- Had trouble remembering recent lectures
- Required extensive notes and review
- Experienced afternoon energy crashes
- Struggled with timed tests despite knowing the material
- Had frequent tension headaches
- Difficulty with physical education despite being "in shape"

The Assessment Revelation

Comprehensive testing revealed:

1. Sleep Architecture Disruption:
   - Fragmented sleep patterns
   - Minimal deep sleep
   - Frequent micro-arousals

- Poor sleep efficiency
2. Breathing Issues:
    - Mouth breathing during sleep
    - Upper airway resistance
    - Low tongue posture
    - Restricted nasal breathing
3. Physical Findings:
    - TMJ tension
    - Neck muscle strain
    - Poor oxygen utilization
    - Elevated cortisol levels

The "But He's Fine" Barrier

The biggest challenge wasn't identifying the problems it was convincing his parents that their high-achieving son could be doing even better. Common responses included:

- "But his grades are perfect"
- "He's more focused than his peers"
- "Everyone's tired in high school"
- "He's just pushing himself to get into a good college"

Breaking Through

What finally convinced them was a simple question: "What if all this success is happening not because of his poor sleep, but in spite of it?"

The Treatment Journey

We implemented a comprehensive approach:

1. Myofunctional therapy to improve tongue position
2. Breathing retraining
3. Sleep hygiene protocols
4. Stress management techniques
5. Gradual caffeine reduction
6. Environmental modifications

Initial Resistance

Michael initially resisted some changes:

- Fear of losing study time
- Worry about academic performance
- Attachment to his routine
- Concern about college applications

The Transformation

Within three months:

- Study time reduced by 2 hours daily
- Test scores improved by 15%
- Memory retention increased dramatically
- Energy drinks no longer needed
- Athletic performance improved
- Headaches resolved
- Time management enhanced
- Public speaking improved
- Creativity flourished

The Surprising Benefits

Unexpected improvements included:

- Enhanced musical ability
- Better emotional regulation
- Improved social relationships
- Increased interest in sports
- More efficient learning
- Better stress management
- Improved problem-solving abilities

The Long-Term Impact

By graduation:

- SAT scores exceeded expectations
- Accepted to top-choice universities

- Developed new interests and hobbies
- Maintained academic excellence with less effort
- Became an advocate for sleep health

Michael's Reflection

During a follow-up visit, Michael shared: "I thought I was performing at my peak before. Now I realize I was operating like a high-end computer with a partially clogged fan still fast, but nowhere near its true potential."

Lessons Learned

Key takeaways from Michael's case:

1. Excellence doesn't equal optimal health
2. High achievement can mask health issues
3. Working harder isn't always the answer
4. Sleep quality affects performance quality
5. Potential is often underestimated

This case revolutionized how I approach high-achieving patients. It taught me that success isn't just about working harder it's about optimizing our body's natural capabilities through proper rest, breathing, and function.

What Was Missed: Poor oxygenation, fragmented REM sleep, and chronic mouth breathing.

What Was Given: Sleep hygiene protocols, nasal breathing therapy, and stress management.

Outcome: Michael's academic performance improved, and he no longer needed caffeine.

The Successful Executive

Maria seemed to have it all great career, beautiful family, but she was barely hanging on. Despite sleeping 8 hours, she was exhausted.

Standard sleep study showed:

- Normal AHI

- Minimal oxygen desaturation
- No significant apneas

But further investigation revealed:

- Upper airway resistance
- Chronic mouth breathing
- Tongue thrust
- Poor sleep architecture
- Getting up 1-3 times a night to pee

After 6 months of treatment:

All the above symptom were gone

- Tongue was no longer blocking the airway
- Mouth breathing stopped
- Tongue thrust was gone
- Better sleep and no longer tired in the morning
- No more waking or getting up at night

The Athlete's Journey: James's Story

The Elite Athlete's Plateau

James was a 28-year-old professional triathlete who had hit a wall in his training. Despite:

- Training 20+ hours weekly
- Perfect nutrition
- Expert coaching
- Recovery protocols
- Optimal heart rate
- Ideal body composition

His performance had plateaued, and his race times were getting slower despite increased training intensity.

The Breaking Point

It wasn't fatigue or injury that brought James to my office it was his girlfriend's complaint about his snoring. "I'm in the best shape of my life," he insisted. "How can I have a breathing problem?"

The Athletic Assessment

Initial examination revealed:

- Forward head posture
- Narrow dental arches
- Restricted nasal breathing
- Tongue-tie
- Teeth wear patterns
- Enlarged tonsils
- Poor tongue posture

Training Impact

His training log showed concerning patterns:

- Inconsistent performance
- Longer recovery needs
- Variable heart rate data
- Decreased speed
- Reduced endurance
- Morning fatigue
- Post-training headaches

Comprehensive Evaluation

Testing uncovered multiple issues:

1. Sleep Architecture:
   - Disrupted deep sleep
   - Limited REM cycles
   - Frequent micro-arousals
   - Poor recovery patterns

2. Breathing Mechanics:
     - ○ Mouth breathing during exercise
     - ○ Inefficient oxygen utilization
     - ○ Restricted nasal airways
     - ○ Poor breathing patterns under stress
3. Performance Metrics:
     - ○ Elevated morning cortisol
     - ○ Delayed recovery markers
     - ○ Compromised HRV scores
     - ○ Reduced testosterone levels
     - ○ Impaired glucose regulation

The Athletic Sleep-Performance Connection

We discovered James was:

- Getting quantity but not quality sleep
- Compensating with increased training
- Creating more stress response
- Reducing recovery capacity
- Limiting performance potential

The Treatment Protocol

We implemented a comprehensive approach:

1. Sleep Optimization:
     - ○ Environment modification
     - ○ Temperature regulation
     - ○ Timing adjustments
     - ○ Recovery protocols
2. Breathing Rehabilitation:
     - ○ Nasal breathing training
     - ○ Tongue position correction
     - ○ Myofunctional therapy
     - ○ Exercise breathing patterns
3. Training Adjustments:
     - ○ Recovery integration

- o Intensity modification
- o Breathing work
- o Sleep priority

The Athletic Challenge

Initially, James resisted:

- Reducing training volume
- Changed breathing patterns
- Sleep schedule adjustments
- Recovery protocols

The Transformation

Within three months:

- Race times improved by 8%
- Recovery time decreased by 40%
- Sleep quality improved dramatically
- Morning HRV increased
- Training consistency improved
- Energy levels stabilized

Performance Improvements

Specific gains:

- Swimming efficiency up by 12%
- Cycling power increased by 15%
- Running economy improved by 10%
- Transition times decreased
- Mental focus sharpened
- Race strategy improved

The Competitive Edge

After six months:

- Personal records broken

- Podium finishes increased
- Injuries decreased
- Training consistency improved
- Recovery optimized
- Performance predictability enhanced

Unexpected Benefits

James also experienced:

- Better stress management
- Improved relationship quality
- Enhanced mental clarity
- Reduced inflammation
- Better immune function
- Improved digestion

Long-Term Impact

One year later:

- Professional ranking improved
- Sponsorship opportunities increased
- Training efficiency optimized
- Life balance achieved
- Career longevity enhanced

The Ripple Effect

James's success influenced:

- Training methodology
- Team protocols
- Coach education
- Athletic community awareness

Key Lessons

This case demonstrated:

1. Elite fitness doesn't equal optimal sleep

2. Breathing affects performance
3. Recovery quality trumps quantity
4. Sleep architecture influences gains
5. Proper breathing enhances endurance

Performance Markers to Monitor

- Morning heart rate
- Recovery rates
- Sleep quality
- Breathing patterns
- Training consistency
- Mental clarity
- Race performance

The New Understanding

James's journey highlighted:

- Sleep's role in peak performance
- Breathing's impact on endurance
- Recovery's importance in progress
- Integration of health systems
- Balance of training and rest

Long-Term Success

Today, James advocates for:

- Sleep quality assessment
- Breathing pattern awareness
- Recovery prioritization
- Holistic training approaches
- Performance integration

This case revolutionized how I approach athletic performance, showing that sometimes the path to peak performance starts with optimal sleep and breathing patterns.

The Chronic Pain Patient: Linda's Journey

A Decade of Pain

Linda, a 45-year-old accountant, had been living with chronic pain for over ten years. Her medical file was thick with diagnoses:

- Fibromyalgia
- Chronic neck pain
- Migraine headaches
- TMJ disorder
- Lower back pain
- Shoulder tension

She'd tried everything:

- Physical therapy
- Chiropractic care
- Massage therapy
- Acupuncture
- Pain medications
- Anti-inflammatory drugs
- Multiple surgeries

The Breaking Point

Linda came to our office not for sleep issues she was there because her teeth were wearing down. "My dentist says I'm grinding my teeth," she explained. "But with all the pain medications I'm on, I didn't think I could be grinding. I sleep like the dead."

The Hidden Connection

During her examination, I noticed:

- Severe tooth wear
- Forward head posture
- Tension in facial muscles
- Dark circles under eyes

- Restricted breathing patterns
- Poor tongue posture
- Morning facial pain
- Frequent sighing

The Sleep Investigation

When we dug deeper, Linda revealed:

- She needed 10+ hours in bed to function
- Woke feeling unrefreshed
- Had morning headaches
- Experienced brain fog
- Required increasing pain medication
- Had dry mouth in the morning
- Frequently woke to use the bathroom
- Partner reported she made "choking sounds"

Comprehensive Assessment

Testing revealed multiple issues:

1. Sleep Architecture:
   - Fragmented sleep patterns
   - Minimal deep sleep
   - Frequent arousals
   - Upper airway resistance
2. Breathing Patterns:
   - Chronic mouth breathing
   - Restricted nasal airways
   - Poor oxygen saturation
   - Shallow breathing habits
3. Physical Findings:
   - Severe tongue tension
   - Restricted airways
   - Postural compensation
   - Muscle dysfunction

The Pain-Sleep Cycle

We discovered Linda was caught in a vicious cycle:

1. Pain disrupted sleep
2. Poor sleep increased inflammation
3. Inflammation increased pain
4. Stress about pain affected sleep
5. Medication side effects impacted breathing
6. Breathing issues fragmented sleep
7. And the cycle continued...

Breaking the Cycle

Our treatment approach focused on:

1. Airway Management:
   - Nasal breathing retraining
   - Tongue position correction
   - Myofunctional therapy
   - Postural alignment
2. Sleep Optimization:
   - Sleep hygiene protocols
   - Breathing exercises
   - Environmental modifications
   - Proper pillow support
3. Pain Management Integration:
   - Coordinated care with pain specialist
   - Gradual medication adjustment
   - Body awareness techniques
   - Stress reduction strategies

The Transformation

Within six months:

- Sleep quality improved dramatically
- Pain levels decreased by 60%

- Medication needs reduced
- Energy levels increased
- Brain fog lifted
- Grinding decreased
- Headaches reduced
- Mood improved

Unexpected Benefits

Linda also experienced:

- Better digestion
- Improved focus
- Enhanced emotional regulation
- Reduced anxiety
- Better work performance
- Improved relationships
- Renewed interest in life

One Year Later

Linda's progress continued:

- Pain medication reduced by 75%
- Sleep normalized to 7-8 hours
- Regular exercise became possible
- Return to social activities
- Career advancement
- Overall life satisfaction improved

The Ripple Effect

Linda's success influenced:

- Her family's sleep habits
- Workplace wellness programs
- Support group awareness
- Healthcare provider education

Key Lessons

Linda's case taught us:

1. Pain management must include sleep assessment
2. Breathing affects pain perception
3. Sleep quality impacts healing
4. Medication effectiveness relates to sleep
5. Holistic approach yields better results

Warning Signs to Watch:

For chronic pain patients:

- Unrefreshing sleep
- Morning pain
- Increasing medication needs
- Daytime fatigue
- Mood changes
- Cognitive decline
- Grinding/clenching

The New Understanding

Linda's journey highlighted how:

- Sleep quality affects pain perception
- Breathing patterns influence pain levels
- Proper rest enables healing
- Body position affects pain
- Sleep architecture influences recovery

Long-Term Impact

Today, Linda advocates for:

- Sleep assessment in pain management
- Breathing awareness
- Comprehensive treatment approaches
- Patient education

- Early intervention

This case revolutionized how I approach chronic pain patients, showing that sometimes the path to pain relief starts with addressing sleep and breathing issues.

> **What Was Missed:** Mouth breathing, fragmented sleep, and airway resistance.

> **What Was Given:** Breathing retraining, tongue posture correction, and sleep hygiene improvements.

> **Outcome:** Within six months, Linda's pain decreased by 60%, and she reduced her medication by 75%.

Professional Guidance

- Consult a Health Coach or Nutritionist: Working with a professional can help personalize your wellness plan and offer guidance tailored to your specific needs.
- Myofunctional Therapy: If you struggle with breathing patterns or oral health issues, consider working with a myofunctional therapist to address these concerns.
- Functional Medicine Practitioners: Chiropractor, OT, PT, and more. These healthcare providers take a holistic, personalized approach to health, focusing on root causes rather than symptoms.

By incorporating practical tips, tools, and resources into your daily routine, you can continue learning and building healthy habits. Whether it's tracking your hydration, practicing mindfulness, or improving your sleep hygiene, staying informed and using the right tools will empower you to take ownership of your health and maintain long-term well-being.

The more I learn the more I know I don't know. I will never stop learning. I will forever be a perpetual student of life. So I am sure I have learned much more since this book was published. I am again very grateful you are reading this book if you made it to the end.

Thank you again for your support.

If I can help, please reach out. I have a free consultation option at www.shereewertz.com

You can follow me on Instagram, linked in, YouTube or my blog www.dentalhygne411.com

I have a course that goes over everything in the book and more. I love to connect and help wherever I can. Health is your greatest wealth.

About the Author

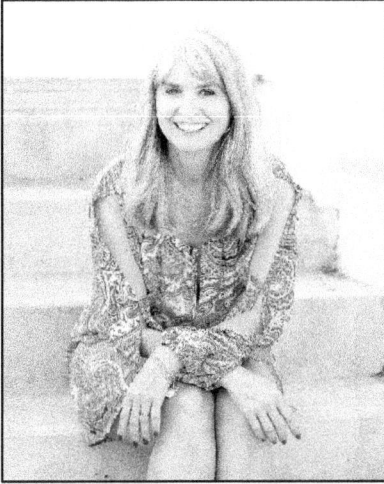

Sheree Wertz is a dedicated dental hygienist, myofunctional therapist, health advocate and educator with a passion for helping people understand the lifelong value of investing in their health. Her journey began with personal health struggles, from iron deficiency to a series of injuries and vision issues as a child, that made learning challenging. Despite these obstacles, she developed an early fascination with oral health a path that would lead her to a rewarding career.

Throughout her life, Sheree faced not only health issues but also significant personal challenges, including overcoming fertility struggles and navigating single parenthood. These experiences taught her the importance of prioritizing one's health, even when life becomes complex. She often reflects on the truth that, while most people will have more than one house or car in their lifetime, they only get one body yet it's often overlooked, with people investing in everything but themselves.

In "O.W.N.E.R." Sheree encourages readers to see their health as their greatest asset. She founded Dental Hygiene 411 to empower professionals, parents and caregivers with the tools and knowledge to make dental health a manageable part of daily life. She works with moms to create child-friendly oral health routines and is passionate about helping other hygienists diversify their careers and protect their livelihoods. Today, she continues to advocate for the essential role of health in living a fulfilling, resilient life. Her work reminds us all that while taking care of ourselves may seem costly, the real price is in neglecting our most valuable asset, our own well-being!

Glossary

Epigenetics

The study of changes in gene expression that do not involve alterations to the DNA sequence itself. Think of it as the "software" that tells your genetic "hardware" how to operate. Lifestyle factors like diet, stress, and sleep can influence your epigenetics, impacting how genes are turned on or off.

Vagus Nerve

A major nerve connecting the brain to the body, playing a critical role in the parasympathetic nervous system, which controls "rest and digest" functions. It helps regulate breathing, heart rate, digestion, and mood, acting as a bridge between your mind and body.

Nasal Hygiene

The practice of maintaining clean and healthy nasal passages to support optimal breathing and prevent issues like congestion or infection. Methods include nasal rinsing, using saline sprays, or ensuring adequate moisture in the air you breathe.

Myofunctional Therapy

A series of exercises designed to improve the function of the muscles in the mouth, face, and throat. It can address issues like mouth breathing, improper swallowing, or snoring by retraining muscle patterns.

Oral Microbiome

The ecosystem of bacteria and microorganisms living in your mouth. A balanced oral microbiome is essential for maintaining oral health, as it helps protect against cavities, gum disease, and other conditions.

Nasal Breathing

The practice of breathing primarily through the nose rather than the mouth. Nasal breathing filters, warms, and humidifies the air, improving oxygen absorption and overall health.

Oxidative Stress

A condition caused by an imbalance between free radicals (unstable molecules) and antioxidants in the body. It can lead to cell damage and contribute to aging and various diseases.

Holistic Health

An approach to wellness that considers the whole mind, mouth, body than focusing on individual symptoms or isolated body systems.

Fight or Flight Response

The body's automatic reaction to perceived danger, activating the sympathetic nervous system. This response increases heart rate, redirects blood to muscles, and prepares the body to either face or escape a threat.

pH Balance

A measure of how acidic or alkaline your body is. A balanced pH supports proper bodily function, including digestion, metabolism, and immune response. The ideal pH of the body is slightly alkaline, around 7.35–7.45.

Tongue Posture

The resting position of the tongue in the mouth. Ideally, the tongue should rest on the roof of the mouth, which supports proper breathing, jaw development, and overall oral health.

Sleep Disordered Breathing (SDB)

A group of conditions, such as sleep apnea and snoring, that affect how you breathe during sleep. These disorders can disrupt sleep quality and impact overall health.

Sympathetic vs. Parasympathetic Nervous System

The sympathetic system is responsible for "fight or flight" responses, while the parasympathetic system manages "rest and digest" activities. Both systems are part of the autonomic nervous system, which controls involuntary body functions.

Genetics vs. Epigenetics

Genetics refers to the DNA you inherit from your parents, while epigenetics refers to how your environment and lifestyle can affect the expression of those genes.

Mind-Mouth-Body Connection

The concept that oral health is deeply connected to overall health.

Appendices

Resources and Further Reading: Recommended books, websites, and tools.

Bibliography

Breathing and Airway Health

1. Nestor, J. (2020). *Breath: The New Science of a Lost Art*. Riverhead Books.
   This book explores the science of breathing and provides actionable insights on improving health through optimal breathing techniques.

2. Dassani, M. (n.d.). *Airway is Life: Waking Up to Your Family's Sleep Crisis*. Focuses on the importance of airway health for family well-being, addressing common sleep and breathing issues.

3. Olsson, A. (2019). *Conscious Breathing: Discover the Power of Your Breath*. Scribe Publications.
   A comprehensive guide on how conscious breathing can impact physical and mental health.

Oral Health and Myofunctional Therapy

1. Moeller, J. L. (n.d.). *Is Your Tongue Killing You? Learn How to Sleep, Breathe, Chew and Swallow Correctly*.
   Offers insights on proper tongue posture and function for improved sleep, breathing, and overall health.

2. Lim, S. (n.d.). *Breathe, Sleep, Thrive*.
   A holistic approach to addressing breathing and sleep issues for optimal growth and **health in children.**

Health, Healing, and Holistic Wellness

1. Hay, L. (1984). *You Can Heal Your Life*. Hay House Inc.
   Explores the mind-body connection, focusing on healing through positive beliefs and lifestyle changes.

2. Passaler, L. (n.d.). *Heal Your Nervous System*.
   This book discusses ways to support and balance the nervous system for overall health and resilience.

3. Murphy, J. (1963). *The Power of Your Subconscious Mind*. Prentice Hall.

Sleep Science and Wellness

1. Walker, M. (2017). *Why We Sleep: Unlocking the Power of Sleep and Dreams*. Scribner.
   Provides a deep dive into the science of sleep, with practical advice for improving sleep quality.
2. Moore, S. (n.d.). *Sleep Wrecked Kids: Helping Parents Restore Their Child's Sleep for a Healthier, Happier Family*.
   Focuses on strategies to address sleep issues in children, emphasizing the role of proper sleep in development.

Nutrition and Diet

1. Clear, J. (2018). *Atomic Habits: An Easy & Proven Way to Build Good Habits & Break Bad Ones*.
   A guide to creating sustainable health routines by building positive habits and breaking negative ones.
2. Gioffre, D. (2018). *Get Off Your Acid: 7 Steps in 7 Days to Lose Weight, Fight Inflammation, and Reclaim Your Health & Energy*. Da Capo Lifelong Books.
   A practical guide for reducing acidity in the body to improve energy and reduce inflammation.
3. Young, R. O., & Young, S. R. (2008). *The pH Miracle: Balance Your Diet, Reclaim Your Health*. Grand Central Life & Style.
   A foundational guide on maintaining an alkaline diet to promote overall health.
4. Vasey, C. (2006). *The Acid-Alkaline Diet for Optimum Health: Restore Your Health by Creating pH Balance in Your Diet*. Healing Arts Press.
   Explores dietary changes for achieving pH balance and supporting wellness.
5. Gates, D. (2003). *The Body Ecology Diet: Recovering Your Health and Rebuilding Your Immunity*. Body Ecology.
   A holistic approach to nutrition, focusing on gut health and immunity.

Gut Health and the Mind-Body Connection

- Mayer, E. A. (2016). *The Mind-Gut Connection: How the Hidden Conversation Within Our Bodies Impacts Our Mood, Our Choices, and Our Overall Health*. Harper Wave.

  Discusses the link between gut health, mental health, and well-being, with practical steps for digestive health.

Websites:

- https://www.theultimatehuman.com/ Gary Brecka
- https://water.usgs.gov/edu/propertyyou.html
- www.burstoralcare.com Use code healthymouth
- https://arogalife.com/en-us/healthymouth/distributor-profile/26092
- https://somnifix.com/blogs/snews/snoring-solution
- https://www.sleepfoundation.org/sleep-aids/side-effects-of-sleeping-pills
- https://link.springer.com/article/10.1007/s10919-010-0098-6
- https://essentialhealthfoods.com.au/how-old-are-your-taste-buds-10-days-to-14-days/